HEALTH CARE IN TRANSITION

THE JOURNEY TO UNIVERSAL HEALTH INSURANCE COVERAGE

WHAT ARE THE LESSONS FOR UGANDA AND THE OTHER LMIC?

HEALTH CARE IN TRANSITION

Additional books and e-books in this series can be found on Nova's website under the Series tab.

HEALTH CARE IN TRANSITION

THE JOURNEY TO UNIVERSAL HEALTH INSURANCE COVERAGE

WHAT ARE THE LESSONS FOR UGANDA AND THE OTHER LMIC?

ROBERT BASAZA
PROSSY KIDDU NAMYALO
CHRISPUS MAYORA
AND
DONALD S. SHEPARD
EDITORS

nova
Medicine & Health
New York

Library of Congress Cataloging-in-Publication Data

Names: Basaza, Robert, editor. | Kiddu Namyalo, Prossy, editor. | Mayora, Chrispus, editor. | Shepard, Donald S., editor.
Title: The journey to universal health insurance coverage : what are the lessons for uganda and the other lmic? / Robert Basaza, editor, Professor of Public Health and Health Economics, St. Augustine, International University, Uganda, Prossy Kiddu Namyalo, editor, Public Health Expert and Lecturer, Ndejje University, Uganda, Chrispus Mayora, editor, Lecturer and Health Economist, Makerere University School of Public Health, Uganda, Donald S. Shepard, editor, Professor at the Schneider Institute for Health Policy, Heller School for Social Policy and Management, Brandeis University, MA, USSeries: Health Care in Transition.
Description: New York : Nova Science Publishers, [2020] | Series: Health care in transition | Includes bibliographical references and index. |
Identifiers: LCCN 2020033931 (print) | LCCN 2020033932 (ebook) | ISBN 9781536183238 (hardcover) | ISBN 9781536184709 (adobe pdf)
Subjects: LCSH: National health insurance--Uganda. | Medical care--Uganda. | National health insurance--Developing countries. | Medical care--Developing countries.
Classification: LCC RA440.55 .U46 2020 (print) | LCC RA440.55 (ebook) | DDC 368.4/20096761--dc23
LC record available at https://lccn.loc.gov/2020033931
LC ebook record available at https://lccn.loc.gov/2020033932

Published by Nova Science Publishers, Inc. † New York

DEDICATION

To all healthcare seekers who failed to receive appropriate services because of lack of money.

To all Ugandan and global promoters of health insurance.

CONTENTS

PREFACE

Access to healthcare is a universal human right and universal health insurance is one of the instruments towards attainment of universal health coverage. Universal health insurance has been proven to reduce catastrophic episodes at the point of receipt of healthcare to millions of households. This book elaborates on the Uganda's Journey to universal health insurance coverage and provides lessons that apply to other LMICs. The book elucidates Uganda's health financing system and details the proposed national health insurance schemes. Besides the local achievements, reference is also made to global success stories of Rwanda, Ghana, Tanzania, China, among others. Practitioners in similar settings will find this book handy in designing or operating appropriate health financing mechanisms. This book will further contribute towards global development of universal health coverage and subsequently ensure healthy lives and promote wellbeing.

Chapter 1 - The opening part of this chapter presents the socio-economic and political profile of Uganda where income and democratic profile, health system delivery and human resources for health are addressed. The second part is on health financing profile in Uganda. In this second part, the current health financing of health services, health protection schemes and free care in government facilities are elaborated. Finally, an implementation status of the Abuja declaration by the country is expounded as follows: Uganda is a low-income country with a Gross National Income (GNI) of US$ 600 per capita in 2013, US $ 660 in 2014, and now at US$ 660 in 2016. The population living below US $1.2 per-day poverty line in 2017 was 27%. The maternal mortality ratio stands at 343 while the under-five mortality rate is at 54.6. The overall literacy rate for persons aged 10 years and above was 72% in 2017. This is coupled with the high fertility rate which at 6.2 per woman and is the second-highest rate in the world. although it dropped slightly to 5.8 children in 2014. The country's health system is pluralistic, with government providing 52% of the healthcare services while the private sector provides 48%. The private sector consists of Private Not for Profit Providers who are largely religious based institutions. On the other hand, the Private For-Profit providers consists of individual owned facilities. Other private providers are traditional and complementary practitioners. Uganda as a country experiences high levels of out-of-pocket expenditure at 40% against WHO recommended level of household out-of-pocket spending on health which is less than 15%. The Per Capita expenditure is US$ 51 with the government health financing accounted for 17% ($10 per capita) of the Current Health Expenditure (CHE). This CHE as a percentage of GDP is 1.3%, against the minimum recommended level of 4% in the HSDP when compared to 6.15% in the African countries. Most notably, in 2001, the Government of Uganda through a presidential decree abolished user fees in government facilities except the private wings in hospitals. Uganda is the only country in East Africa with no contributory social health insurance scheme. There are 26 community-based health insurance schemes with the majority in the southern part of the country and total enrollment is 150,000 people. There are private commercial health insurance schemes covering 700,000 people. The government still faces the policy challenge of increasing health expenditure as a proportion of public financing from the current 7% to meet the Abuja target of 15%.

Chapter 2 - Using data from the literature, documents, and interviews with stakeholders, this study which was commissioned by USAID Uganda, examined the cost-effectiveness of reproductive health vouchers (RHVs) and subsidy of community-based health insurance to improve maternal outcomes in Uganda. According to World Health Organization, a service is considered highly cost effective if it can generate a disability adjusted life year (DALY) at a cost below the country's gross domestic product (GDP) per capita [1, 2]. The study found that both vouchers and community-based health insurance (CBHI) are highly cost-effective. At most likely costs of US$302 per DALY averted for vouchers and $309 for subsidy of CBHI. both interventions are highly cost-effective and virtually identical in their cost-effectiveness ratios. Both cost-effectiveness ratios are below US$510, Uganda's GDP per capita. On policy grounds, the subsidy of CBHI is more consistent with a broader policy supported by Uganda and other partner states in the East African community of expanding social health protection through enrolling the population in universal health insurance. Insurance should also include outreach to encourage poor women to deliver at health facilities, transportation to and from health centers for deliveries, and incentives to health workers for increased volume and improved quality. In the neighboring country of Rwanda, with a health system like that of Uganda offering government, non-government, or faith-based health facilities, such incentives proved successful in improving use of primary care services. Insurance models that create sustainable incentives for providers to offer quality care have the potential to increase access through partnerships between care providers and member groups or CBHI plans. This chapter is an update from the original text presented to the Ugandan Health Sector in 2015.

Chapter 3 - The paper aims at presenting the genesis and development of Community Based Health Insurance (CHI) and contributing knowledge to the development of universal health insurance in Uganda, a key strategy under universal health coverage in sustainable development goals. A cross sectional descriptive and retrospective study of CHI schemes in Uganda was done. Data was obtained through the records of the CHI umbrella organization; Uganda Community Based Health Financing Association. Data extraction sheets were developed and used to analyze individual scheme records. This was complemented by literature review on CHI in Uganda, the region and beyond. A majority of the schemes are found in Southern and Western Uganda with a few in the Central region. The Eastern and the Northern Districts are starting to form them. Currently, there is no regulatory instrument for CHIS but they are registered as either community-based organizations at district level or non-government organizations by the Registrar of Companies at national level. The community managed CHIs have majority of the beneficiaries. A comparative case study about Rwanda with a rather successful case and larger coverage (over 75% of Rwandas' 10 million people) is presented. CHI schemes were started with donor support and do not have a legal framework for the last 22 years. They face several challenges such as poverty of the population, limited government buy-in and inadequate technical capacity by the promoters. This has affected expansion of the schemes both in enrolment and depth of the package. The schemes face a policy dilemma of promotion of contributory payment for healthcare amidst a policy of free healthcare by government. The future of CHI will depend on the design of the proposed National Health Insurance and the will of the political actors in Uganda to establish a prepayment system in line with other East African Community Partner States.

Chapter 4 - Health cooperatives are an important solution to health care challenges in developing countries because they incentivize members to seek care early and providers to keep members healthy and improve quality of care. The purpose of this chapter is to provide strategies and lessons learnt from cooperative health financing in Uganda in order to enable health stakeholders to increase access to care while improving health outcomes. This chapter also aims at helping governments in similar context to design efficient and effective universal health care systems. Methods: The sources of literature have been performance reports from HealthPartners Uganda and USA and published literature from similar schemes. The authors and institutional experience have been used to identify and pull literature and other relevant information on this topic. Discussion and lessons for the health sector: Studies show that in addition to seeking care sooner, health cooperative members in Uganda adopted more preventive healthy behaviors like washing hands and sleeping under long lasting insecticide treated mosquito nets compared to non-members. Providers who offer cooperative services enjoyed increased cost recovery due to reduced bad debt. The member-owned structure empowered beneficiaries to take control of their health and to demand quality services from their care providers. Conclusion:

By applying these lessons, governments can avoid common pitfalls and scale up systems to benefit all stakeholders with a focus on the informal sector as part of broader national health insurance scheme.

Chapter 5 - Uganda is the last East African country to adopt a National Health Insurance Scheme (NHIS). In order to lessen the inequitable burden of healthcare spending, health financing reform has focused on the establishment of national health insurance. The objective of this investigation was to depict how stakeholders and their power and interests have shaped the process of agenda setting and policy formulation for Uganda's proposed NHIS. The study provides a contextual analysis of the development of NHIS policy within the context of national policies and processes. The methodology is a single case study of agenda setting and policy formulation related to the proposed NHIS in Uganda. It involves an analysis of the real-life context, the content of proposals, the process, and a retrospective stakeholder analysis in terms of policy development. Data collection comprised a literature review of published documents, technical reports, policy briefs, and memos obtained from Uganda's Ministry of Health and other unpublished sources. Formal discussions were also held with ministry staff involved in the design of the scheme and some members of the task force in order to obtain clarification, verify events, and gain additional information. The process of developing the NHIS has been an incremental one, characterized by small-scale, gradual changes and repeated adjustments through various stakeholder engagements during the four phases of development: from 1995 to 1999; 2000 to 2005; 2006 to 2011 and 2011 to-date. In spite of political will and government buy-in, progress with the NHIS has been slow, more less like an unwinding river in mountainous gauge and is yet to be implemented. Stakeholders, notably the private sector, played an important role in influencing the pace of the development process and the currently proposed design of the scheme. This study underscores the importance of stakeholder analysis in major health reforms. Early use of stakeholder analysis combined with an ongoing review and revision of NHIS policy proposals during stakeholder discussions would be an effective strategy for avoiding potential pitfalls and obstacles in policy implementation. Given the private sector's influence on negotiations over health insurance design in Uganda, this paper also reviews the experiences of two countries with similar stakeholder dynamics.

Chapter 6 - Introduction: Uganda since 2006, has been in the process of drafting a National Health Insurance Scheme Act. At the beginning of drafting the process, Private Commercial Health Insurance (PCHI) was one of the components and was later dropped in the current May 2019 edition of the bill. Persons that are not in formal employment and they don't want to join community health insurance will be enrolled in the PCHI. Methods: The methodology used is descriptive and included reviewing of records from a number of institutions including Uganda Insurers Association, Insurance Regulatory Authority, Health Maintenance Organizations (HMOs), Association among others. Records were supplemented with literature on PCHI in Uganda and other countries, and the authors used both published and grey literature. Findings and Discussion: Majority of the PCHI are employer-based schemes and 75% of the schemes have their own facilities, with the remaining schemes run by insurance companies. These schemes target private formal sector workers and their dependents. Very few members join as individual families. The formal sector is easy to enroll in and can afford relatively higher premiums compared to the rural informal sector workers. There were nine (9) paid up HMOs with a gross written premium (GWP) of UGX 52,159,269,966 in 2016. Currently there are 7 Health Insurance Organizations registered by the Insurance Regulatory Authority. The HIOs operate with a more open access network of providers and generally charge higher premiums than the HMOs. Their costs are likely to be higher since they do not own their own facilities. In the past, insurance services were considered to be a luxury as it was assumed that only the rich people could afford the high premiums. This led to low penetration levels in country. Besides, due to high poverty levels, private health insurance is not well consumed. Private health insurance by nature is costly and only a certain proportion of the population may afford it. Depending on how many lives an insurer has on the schemes, extrapolating these figures to total cost shows that this is not a profit driven market because of the high loss ratios. The challenges and lessons learnt are explained in this chapter. In addition, the chapter presents three case studies on specific companies in the business of PCHI.

Chapter 7 - Background**:** Universal health insurance coverage has been proven to reduce catastrophic episodes of health care at the point of delivery to millions of households. Following the health care delivery and access challenge, Ghana established its National Health Insurance Scheme (NHIS) in 2003 with the passing of the National Health Insurance bill into law (Act 650, 2003). The main goal of the NHIS was a pro-poor health financing policy intervention to provide health care to all residents of the country. Since its establishment, the NHIS has achieved a steady growth of up to 41% population coverage in 2016, but with equity and financial sustainability challenges. The authors present detailed pathways of the health financing reform and universal health insurance in Ghana. Purpose: This chapter presents the detailed experience of Ghana's health care financing pathways, the challenges, the best practices and lessons learned for possible replication in the establishment of Universal Health Insurance in Uganda and other similar settings. Methods: This paper used mixed methods approach. The authors conducted an extensive desk review of relevant literature about Ghana's NHIS, 12 in-depth interviews with selected healthcare providers, 20 in-depth interviews and focus group discussions with key personnel and management of the National Health Insurance Authority, Ministry of Health, and Ghana Health Services. Findings: The study revealed very useful lessons in political economy of health financing in Ghana, the implementation processes, and governance, equity and sustainability challenges of the NHIS. Appropriate legislation, social solidarity, strong political will, tax funding and safety net for the poor and vulnerable are necessary determinants of a successful NHIS. Adopting appropriate principles such as solidarity, cross-subsidization, equity and empowerment of insured members to have a voice in the scheme and avoiding excessive domestic politicization of a health insurance scheme can effectively enhance its success. The study also found that adopting fee-for-service payment method without effective control measures can be a recipe for healthcare provider fraud. However, the capitation payment method engenders shared responsibilities between the provider, the purchaser and the patients, hence a triple win, when implemented with effective monitoring mechanisms. Finally, while the study found generous health insurance benefits package, and premium exemptions for the vulnerable as cardinal principles of a pro-poor health insurance scheme, the paradox is that these same measures, if not effectively managed, can increase the costs of the NHIS and cause its collapse. Conclusion: The Ghana's NHIS model shows that countries do not need huge resources or a gold standard plan before establishing a universal health insurance scheme. With a combination of appropriate legislation, and tax funding mechanism coupled with strong political will, a national health insurance scheme can be established using the learning by doing approach while adopting corrective measures on its path to success. This Ghana NHIS model is a practical example for replication in other developing, and even advanced countries. These lessons learned from Ghana's NHIS could serve as guiding principles for Uganda and the rest of the East African Community in their quest for universal health insurance schemes.

Chapter 8 - This Chapter focuses on the possible ways forward with health financing and establishment of universal health insurance coverage in Uganda. It also provides what LMICs with similar level of development like Uganda could consider for adoption. A measured quantity, quality and types of reforms may be necessary.

ACKNOWLEDGMENTS

The editors wish to thank all chapter authors, reviewers and other persons who made the writing and publishing of this book possible.

In: The Journey …
Editors: Robert Basaza et al.
ISBN: 978-1-53618-323-8

Chapter 1

HEALTH FINANCING IN UGANDA: HOW IS UGANDA RESPONDING TO ABUJA DECLARATION?

***Robert Basaza*[1,*], *Prossy K. Namyalo*[3], *David Ogubi*[2], *Grace Kabaniha*[3] and *Chrispus Mayora*[4]**

[1]Gudie Incubation Centre, Kira Municipality Uganda
and Uganda Christian University Mukono, MPHL Program
[2]International Health Sciences University, Uganda
[3]Ndejje University, Faculty of Social Sciences, Uganda
[4]WHO Uganda Country Office
[5]Makerere University School of Public Health, Uganda

ABSTRACT

The opening part of this chapter presents the socio-economic and political profile of Uganda where income and democratic profile, health system delivery and human resources for health are addressed. The second part is on health financing profile in Uganda. In this second part, the current

* Corresponding Author's E-mail: rbasaza@gmail.com.

health financing of health services, health protection schemes and free care in government facilities are elaborated. Finally, an implementation status of the Abuja declaration by the country is expounded as follows: Uganda is a low-income country with a Gross National Income (GNI) of US$ 600 per capita in 2013, US $ 660 in 2014, and now at US$ 660 in 2016. The population living below US $1.2 per-day poverty line in 2017 was 27%. The maternal mortality ratio stands at 343 while the under-five mortality rate is at 54.6. The overall literacy rate for persons aged 10 years and above was 72% in 2017. This is coupled with the high fertility rate which at 6.2 per woman and is the second-highest rate in the world. Although it dropped slightly to 5.8 children in 2014. The country's health system is pluralistic, with government providing 52% of the healthcare services while the private sector provides 48%. The private sector consists of Private Not for Profit Providers who are largely religious based institutions. On the other hand, the Private For-Profit providers consists of individual owned facilities. Other private providers are traditional and complementary practitioners.

Uganda as a country experiences high levels of out-of-pocket expenditure at 40% against WHO recommended level of household out-of-pocket spending on health which is less than 15%. The Per Capita expenditure is US$ 51 with the government health financing accounted for 17% ($10 per capita) of the Current Health Expenditure (CHE). This CHE as a percentage of GDP is 1.3%, against the minimum recommended level of 4% in the HSDP when compared to 6.15% in the African countries. Most notably, in 2001, the Government of Uganda through a presidential decree abolished user fees in government facilities except the private wings in hospitals. Uganda is the only country in East Africa with no contributory social health insurance scheme. There are 26 community-based health insurance schemes with the majority in the southern part of the country and total enrollment is 150,000 people. There are private commercial health insurance schemes covering 700,000 people. The government still faces the policy challenge of increasing health expenditure as a proportion of public financing from the current 7% to meet the Abuja target of 15%.

ABBREVIATIONS

CBHI	Community Based Health Insurance;
CHE	Current Health Expenditure;
LMIC	Low and Middle-Income Countries;
GDP	Gross Domestic Product;
HSDP	Health Sector Development Plan;

MOHU	Ministry of Health Uganda;
NHIS	National Health Insurance Scheme;
PCHI	Private Commercial Health Insurance;
PNFP	Private Not for Profit;
SDG	Sustainable Development Goals;
UCBHFA	Uganda Community Based Health Financing Association;
OOP	Out of Pocket;
WHO	World Health Organization.

INTRODUCTION

This chapter is divided in two parts: Part one provides the socio-economic and political profile of Uganda where income and democratic profile, health system delivery and human resources for health are addressed. Part two is on health financing profile: In this part, the current financing of health services, the health protection schemes and free care in government facilities in Uganda are elaborated and finally an implementation status of the Abuja declaration by the country is explicated.

Socio-Economic and Political Profile of Uganda

Uganda is a low-income country with a Gross National Income (GNI) of US$ 600 Per capita as was in 2013, US $ 660 in 2014, and at US$ 660 in 2016 [1 & 2]. The country's economy remains rural and agrarian with a large proportion of the population still relying on low-paying jobs in the agriculture sector. About three-quarters of Uganda's adult population are employed, mainly in subsistence/peasant farming. The proportion of the population employed in the informal sector was 54.5%, ranking the lowest in the East African (EA) region with 18.4% of the population urbanized in 2014 [3, 4 & 7]. Uganda's economic growth rate has averaged about 5.6% per annum over the past 5 years [5]. This is an indicator of slowing when compared to the 2000–10 period, when Uganda experienced an annual average economic growth of 7% [4]. Nonetheless, an estimated 24.5% of the population was living below the $1.2 per-day poverty line in 2000 and eventually fell to 19.7% in 2015 then rose to 27% in 2016 with more households becoming impoverished as a result of health expenditure on a daily basis [3, 4 & 6].

Maternal mortality ratio stands at 343 while the under-five mortality rate is at 54.6/1000 live births [6] with their percentage diminutions threatening the targets of 54% and 63% respectively for the period between 1990 and 2013 [8 & 9]. Lack of financial access to health services results to poor health and high disease burden of the poor people who have been identified as drivers of poverty in Uganda [9]. This demonstrates the importance of minimizing the financial barriers to health services. It's worthy noting that a large part of the population (86%) resides within a 5-km radius of a health facility and universal primary and secondary education has boosted literacy rates in the country. The overall literacy rate for persons aged 10 years and above was 72% in 2017. Progress in overall human development indicators in the country has been consistent but relatively low. The life expectancy improved from 48.1 years in 1991 to 50.4 years in 2002 and 63.3 years in 2014 [2, 4 & 10]. At the moment, Uganda faces a quadruple epidemic transition of communicable and non-communicable diseases, injuries and maternal, neonatal and child mortalities. Communicable diseases account for 54% of the total burden of disease in the country, with HIV/AIDS, Tuberculosis, and malaria being the leading causes of ill health. Non-communicable diseases are an emerging problem with costly treatment implications. Injuries form 4.8% of hospital-based morbidity. This coupled with the high fertility rate, which is at 5.4 per woman and is the second-highest rate in the world although it dropped slightly to 5.8 among children in 2014. In addition, significant disparities exist in health status among regions and socio-economic strata, with rural areas having the highest burden of ill health and death [4 & 11]. On the political front, Uganda is a Republic and has progressed towards a multiparty democracy with an Executive President [21].

Healthcare System Delivery in Uganda

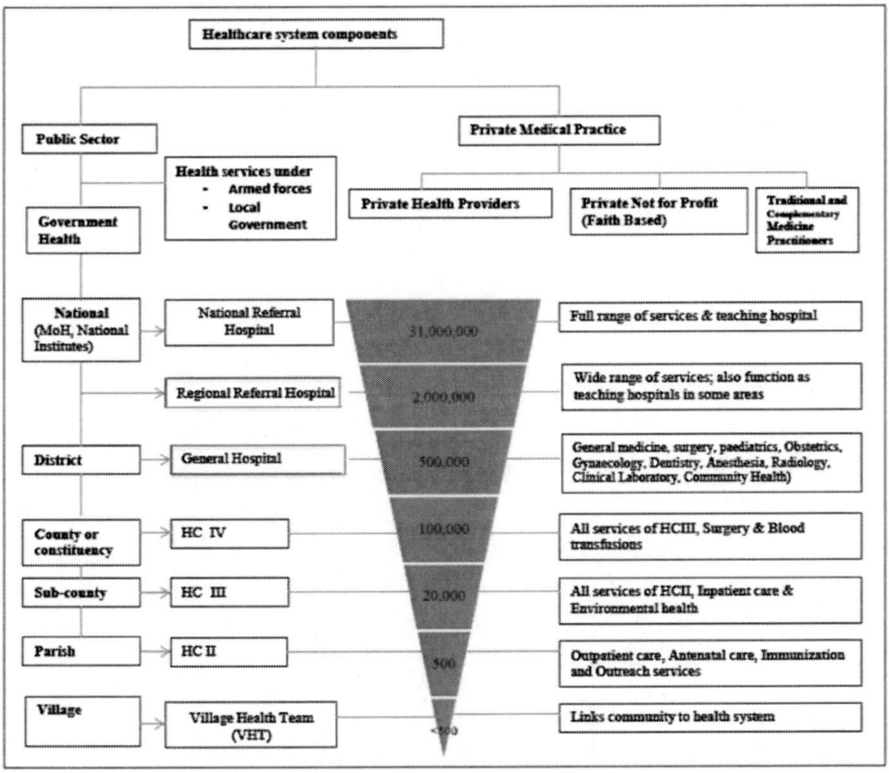

Source: Ministry of Health (2017), Planning Department

Figure 1. Structure of the Healthcare Delivery in Uganda

The Health Sector Development Plan (HSDP) 2015/16-19/20 and the previous Health Sector Strategic and Investment Plan 2010/11-2014/15 underscores the restructuring of the organization and management of the Ministry of Health and the District Health System. They aim to ensure an effective harmony and linkages between the centre and the districts in addition to public and private components. It further calls for the establishment of "a network of functional, efficient and sustainable health infrastructure for effective health care delivery closer to the people." The country's health system is pluralistic with government providing 52% of the healthcare services while the private sector provides 48%. The private sector consists of Private Not for Profit providers who are largely religious based institutions. On the other hand, the Private For Profit providers consist of individual owned facilities. Other private providers are traditional and complementary practitioners [11, 12 & 13]. Service delivery is organized in different levels and functions while responsibilities of each level of the delivery system have been defined. Minimum service standards and staffing levels have been set for each tier of service delivery. The national health delivery system is organized as shown in Figure 1.

Human Resource

Uganda is among the countries in critical need of more health workers to deliver a standard package of health services to the population. The country has 3,692 active doctors providing health care mainly in urban areas with 80% concentrated in cities while the nurses are estimated at 36,031 and with the majority in urban areas [14]. The ratio of providers to population is 1:24,725 and 1:18000 for doctors and nurses respectively (15). According to WHO, a country with less than 2.28 health workers (doctors, nurses and midwives) per 1000 people is regarded to be in severe shortage of health workers to meet its health needs. For Uganda, this ratio was 1:22 in 2006 and about 1:50 in 2013 [9, 11 & 14].

HEALTH FINANCING LANDSCAPE

The Country experiences high levels of Out-of-Pocket expenditure at 40% which does not protect households from catastrophic spending. WHO recommended level of household out of pocket spending on health is 15%. This is in line with World Health Assembly resolution of 2005 on universal coverage and sustainable health financing as well as revisiting the Paris Declaration that calls for greater Investments in the Health Sector. The five-year Health Sector Development Plan (HSDP) recommended a minimum of $73 per capita in the year 2015/16. The recommended per capita health expenditure is a minimum of $84 per capita for low income countries when a country is to increase access to health care and improve quality of services. With the current Ugandan epidemiological profile, relative to the country's desired level of health status, the per capita expenditure of US$ 51 may not move the country towards achieving the Sustainable Development Goals (SDGs). The government health financing accounted for 15% ($11 per capita) of the Current Health Expenditure (CHE). This CHE as a percentage of GDP was 1.4%, as against the minimum recommended level of 4% in the HSDP [11 & 16] and compared to 6.15% in the African countries [17].

Generally, health sector financing in Uganda is a project and vertically oriented, with low investments in overall systems improvement. The incidence of catastrophic health expenditure among the poor steadily increased from 8% in1996 to 28% in 2006 despite the abolition of user fees, which was partly due to the greater use of private providers by the poor [18,19 & 20]. Another factor was frequently unavailability of medicines in public facilities, requiring patients to pay higher prices to acquire medicines at private pharmacies [18, 19, 20 & 21]. Other than revenue collected through taxation and budget support, there is no any other resource-pooling mechanism at the national level. The Private commercial health insurance schemes are mandated by the Insurance Regulatory Authority (IRA) to reinsure the collected premiums and have reserves. In regard to Community based health insurance schemes, the schemes lack a pooling mechanism except for the Save for Health supported schemes in greater Bushenyi and Luwero districts that have district pools and district representatives [8].

Social Health Protection Schemes

The health sector is responsible for social health protection in the country but within the broader framework of social protection (Figure 2).

Social health protection/ Insurance Schemes	Year created	Oversight	Premium	Co-payment	Population Targeted
NHIS	In process of being created	Not yet operational	Not yet operational	Not yet operational	Formal sector
Private health commercial insurance schemes	1994	Collective bargaining by trade unions		Variable and not available to researchers	Formal and informal sector
CBHI	First schemes around 1995. Existence of 26schemes	Community or Private –Not for Profit		up to 20%	rural, poor
Military and • Have their own health centers • Free care when on duty • OOP for specialized treatment	Since Government's existence	Ministries for Defense and One for Internal Affairs	Free care	None	Military and Police

Source: Reference [8]

Figure 2. Health protection schemes in Uganda

Free Care in Government Facilities

In 2001, the Government of Uganda through a Presidential decree abolished user fees in government facilities except the private wings in hospitals; a result of the recognition that user fees were a barrier to the poor utilizing health services. Free care is also accessed in uniformed services such as the military, prisons and police facilities for the disciplined forces and their dependents totaling about 700,000 people [8 &19]. It is not for the entire population and covers for only services available in these units. Payment for services, under staffing, poor infrastructure and inadequate funding remain the major challenges in the private health sector. Other additional issues are: some segment of the population does not believe in free care and there are under the table payments [18 & 22].

Government Subsidy and Donations to Private Health Providers

The government provides subsidies through the public – private partnership which is about 10% to 20% of their operational costs. This has enabled PNFPS to lower user- fees. Social health protection forms are an integral part of the PNFP principles of protecting the poor and other vulnerable populations. Additionally, some private for-profit providers receive government subsidies like funding and salaries for some of the health facility staff as a compensation for provision of select free public health services like immunization [11, 12 & 24].

Community Based Health Insurance Schemes

Community-based health insurance (CBHI) schemes were first created in 1995 in Kisiizi Hospital. There are 26 schemes with the majority in the southern part of the country. The south has relatively better built solidarity structures and higher income compared to the rest of the country. Most schemes operate in PNFPs facilities and have an umbrella organization, Uganda Community Based Health Financing Association (UCBHFA) [7]. Services offered are only those available at the contracted facilities and exclude referral and portability. Even in those areas where CBHI exist, the poor are not subsidized and the premium is still considered expensive [8]. There is no specific legislation or regulatory instruments covering the operations of CBHI. Most of the schemes have changed from facility ownership and are currently owned and managed by the community. The schemes target individual families within existing social groups like burial ceremonies, farmers' groups and schools. They cover about 5%-10% of the population where they are located. They are micro insurance schemes and the total enrollment in the country is 150,000 people [7 & 8]. There is a co-payment for both in and out-patient care which is up to 20% of the health care bill. The schemes target the rural poor who have some income to pay the premium. Those who cannot afford to pay the premium are excluded. Women, children and the elderly who can afford the premium are included. The schemes lack a mechanism of enrolling the indigent who form 19.7% of the population. The challenges of the schemes include: lack of a legal framework, availability of free care in government facilities, poor quality of care which is mainly at hospitals (no gate keeping), poor understanding of insurance principles by the population including politicians at all levels and scheme managers, poverty, lack of trust in leaders, poor design (60% of a group must join as a measure against adverse selection,) and no portability of benefits [7, 23 & 25].

Private Commercial Health Insurance (PCHI) Schemes

The first scheme, the African Air Rescue (AAR) was started in 1994. The majority are employer based schemes of which75% have their own facilities, while the remaining are run by insurance companies. These schemes target private formal sector workers and their dependents. Very few members join as individual families. The formal sector is easy to enroll and can afford relatively higher premiums compared to the rural informal sector workers. They enroll children over three months, exclude the elderly (over 65years of age unless previously enrolled) and cover about 1% of the population mainly in urban areas. They face major challenges like lack of tariffs and rates in Ugandan health care systems (providers charge the amount they want), weak regulation and poor quality of care. Both CBHI and PCHIs do not cover immunization, treatment for HIV or Tuberculosis because they are provided free by vertical government programs. The quality of care for both scheme and non-scheme patients is the same. Patients are only identified at the point of payment [22 & 26].

Other Informal Community Health Insurers

The country has informal community health insurers like funeral groups which also lend money for health care and transportation of the sick like "Engozi." They are localized, small in scale and voluntary. Furthermore, there is family assistance where family members contribute money for the care of their kin who is sick. Like all small homogenous entities, they are unable to diversify risk across the population and are susceptible to adverse selection [25 & 26].

Proposed National Health Insurance Scheme

The Health Sector Development Plan 2015/16-2019/20 points out that the introduction of the National Health Insurance Scheme (NHIS) scheme is one of the health financing interventions to mitigate the high OOP [11]. The design of the scheme is across the government divide and is being spearheaded by the Ministry of Health and will initially target coverage for people in formal employment. The scheme will require both the employee and the employer to each contribute 4% of the employee's salary thus making 8% with no co-payments. The scheme will begin with 10% of the national population (formally employed and their dependents) and later expand to cover the whole population. The informal sector will be required to pay a prescribed premium which has not been decided. Though the scheme is supposed to be an autonomous organization, currently there is lack of capacity in the Ministry of Health to design the scheme [8, 21, 27 & 28]. Other challenges to the proposed scheme are: abolition of user fees in Government units and poor quality of care in both private and public units. NHIs are one of proposed practical instruments towards universal coverage [8 & 28].

Uganda has been with an agenda to develop health insurance as alternative to tax-based financing of health services since 1987. This was a recommendation of the policy review commission which was set up after the civil war [29]. In 2001, Uganda contracted Harvard and Makerere University (in Uganda) Schools of Public Health to carry out a feasibility study on development of social health insurance which informed the design process of the proposed NHIS [28]. The Ministry of Health obtained the certificate of financial implications from Ministry for Finance in 2017. The impact assessment of the Bill was carried out and subsequently, the bill was tabled in Cabinet and passed. Since early 2020, the bill has been before the Health Committee of Parliament. It awaits approval before it is presented in Parliament [35].

There is no one stop reference material to why this East African country has stayed without a specific health insurance agenda and more so why attempts have universal health insurance coverage have not yielded substantial progress. No attempts have been made to elaborate why other East African Countries have national health insurance schemes and Uganda does not have one. This book will fill this vacuum and provide insights for future health insurance development processes in Uganda and related African countries. It will also provide lessons to countries with similar setting and serve as a resource to researchers and scientists in this field.

In regards to lessons from other Low and Middle-Income Countries (LMIC), Uganda stands to benefit from the practical lessons of putting up and running universal health insurance scheme/coverage. Uganda shall also provide lessons to countries considering the same path or on the same path of universal health insurance that face similar circumstances.

How Is Uganda Responding to Abuja Declaration?

Uganda just like the other African states pledged to commit at least 15% of its annual budget to health in 2001. Since, then this target has never been met with the highest of all time being 9.7% in the FY 2004/05. The percentage of the total government budget allocated to the health sector reduced from 9.6% in 2009/2010 [16, 28, 29 & 30] to 8.7% in 2016/17 and 6.4% in 2017/2018 [31 & 37]. The high level task force on innovative international financing for health systems emphasized at least US$ 44 per capita in 2009 and later on US$ 84 in 2017 for provision of key health services for low income countries like Uganda. However, this is far from being met with the current over all per capita health expenditure of US$ 51 with government contributing US$ 10 per capita per annum. This is also still below the Health Sector Development Plan (HSDP) target of US$ 73 per capita in the year 2015/16 [12, 16 & 17].

RESPONSE TO ABUJA DECLARATION BY OTHER AFRICAN COUNTRIES

In this chapter, we do argue that there is no single health financing mechanism that can provide for healthcare alone; the government funding still remains the main source. The other mechanisms can only supplement government efforts to adequately finance health services. This is the same argument advanced by Kutzin et al. in the work on implementing health financing reform [32 & 34]. As the Ugandan health sector makes continued efforts in designing the scheme, the current government still faces the policy challenge of increasing health expenditure. The proportion of public financing from the current 7% to meet the Abuja target of 15% is a milestone to reach. There are only four countries in the continent which were able to meet the 15% target in 2014. These countries are: Gambia, Ethiopia, Swaziland and Malawi [32, 33 & 36].

REFERENCES

[1] The World Bank. 2015. *World Development Indicators 2015*. Washington, DC: World Bank.

[2] The World Bank. 2016. *The Uganda Poverty Assessment Report 2016*. Washington DC, the World Bank Group.

[3] Uganda Bureau of Statistics. 2014. *Statistical Abstract*. Kampala: Uganda Bureau of Statistics.

[4] Uganda Bureau of Statistics. 2015. *Uganda Population and Housing Census Report*. Kampala, UBOS.

[5] Trading Economics. 2017. *Uganda's economic growth rate*. https://tradingeconomics.com/uganda/gdp (Last accessed on 21st June, 2020).

[6] World Health Organization. 2017. *World Health Statistics: Monitoring Health for SDGs*. Geneva, World Health Organization.

[7] *Uganda Community-Based Health Financing Association: Path to Better Health. 2015*. www.ucbhfa.org (last accessed on 10th October 2017).

[8] East African Community. 2014. *Situational Analysis and Feasibility Study of Options for Harmonization of Social Health Protection Systems towards Universal Health Coverage in the East African Community Partner States*. Arusha, Tanzania.

[9] World Health Organisation. 2015. *World Health Statistics*. Geneva: World Health Organisation.

[10] Ministry of Finance Planning and Economic Development. 2002. *Uganda Participatory Poverty Assessment Process (UPPAP)*. Kampala, MFPED.

[11] Ministry of Health. 2015. *Health Sector Development Plan 2015/16-2019/20.* Kampala, Ministry Of Health Uganda.

[12] Ministry of Health. 2010: *Health Sector Development Plan 2015/16-2019/20*. Kampala, Ministry Of Health Uganda.

[13] Ministry of Health. 2017. Online Publications. Website: (Last accessed on 15th December 2017). http://health.go.ug.

[14] Ministry of Health. 2015. Human Resources for Health Bi-Annual Report: *"Improving HRH Evidence for Decision Making*." Kampala, MOHU.

[15] Ministry of Health. 2017. *Annual Health Sector Performance Report 2016/17.* Kampala, Ministry Of Health Uganda.

[16] Ministry Of Health-Uganda. 2017. *Uganda Health Accounts: National Health Expenditure*. Kampala: Ministry Of Health Uganda.

[17] World Health Organization. 2017. Website: *WHO Global Health Expenditure Atlas* (Last accessed on 15th December 2014). http://www.who.int/health-accounts/atlas2014.pdf.

[18] Okuonzi AS. 2004. Learning from failed health reform in Uganda. *BMJ Education and debate*: Vol 329: 13(1173-6).

[19] Orem, N. J. et al. 2011. Abolition of user fees: the Uganda paradox. *Health Policy and Planning* (online). 26(supplementary 2), (Accessed 20th November 2017), pp ii41-1151. Available from: http://heapol.oxfordjournals.org/content/26/suppl_2/ii41.abstract.

[20] Orem, N. J and M. C. Zikusooka. 2010. Health financing reforms in Uganda: How equitable is the proposed National Health Insurance Scheme. *International Journal for Equity in Health* (online). 9(23), (Accessed 20th November 2017), pp. 1-8. Available from: http://www.equityhealthj.com/content/9/1/23.

[21] Basaza, R, T. Cornell and I. Chapcokova. 2013. The players and the processes behind the National Health Insurance Scheme: A case study of Uganda. *BMC Health Services Research*. 13:57.

[22] Providing for Health. 2010: *Health Financing Reform & Social Health Protection, Specifying the options; Follow up visit and dialogue between Ugandan Stakeholders and a P4H Team*. Providing for Health. Uganda: Republic of Uganda.

[23] Save for Health Uganda. 2014. *Annual Report 2013*. Kampala, SHU.

[24] Ministry of Health. 2013. *The Private Public Partnership Health Policy*. Kampala. Ministry Of Health Uganda.

[25] Basaza, KR, Criel B and Stuyft Van der V. 2007. Low enrolment in Ugandan Community Health Insurance Schemes: Underlying causes and policy implications. *BMC Health Services Research,* 7:105.

[26] IRA, 2016, *Personal Communication from Insurance Regulatory Authority of Uganda.*

[27] Ministry of Health. 2019. *The Health Insurance Bill*. Kampala, Ministry of Health Uganda.

[28] Ministry of Health. 2001. *Feasibility analysis of Social Health Insurance in Uganda.* Kampala, Ministry Of Health Uganda.

[29] Ministry of Health. 1987. *Health Policy Review Commission*. Kampala, Ministry Of Health Uganda.

[30] Ministry of Health. 2014. *Annual Health Sector Performance Report 2013/14.* Kampala, Ministry Of Health Uganda.

[31] Ministry of Finance Planning and Economic Development. 2016. *Background to the budget -2016/2017*. Kampala, MFPED.

[32] *Organization of African Unity Abuja declaration on HIV/AIDS, tuberculosis, and other related infectious diseases* (OAU/SPS/ABUJA/3). http://www.un.org/ga/aids/pdf/abuja_declaration.pdf. (Last accessed on 15th December 2017).

[33] Ocampo, AR. 2013. *Health funding in Africa: How close is the AU to meeting Abuja targets? 2017*. Website. https://www.devex.com/news/health-funding-in-africa-how-close-is-the-au-to-meeting-abuja-targets-81567 (Last accessed on 15th December 2017).

[34] World Health Organization (2011. *Abuja Declaration: Ten Years On.* Geneva, World Health Organization.

[35] Ministry of Health, 2017, *Communication from Planning Department of Ministry of Health Uganda and a National Community Health Financing Conference.*

[36] World Health Organization (2017) *Personal communication from WHO Afro Office.*

[37] Ministry of Health. 2018. *Annual Health Sector Performance Report 2017/18.* Kampala, Ministry of Health Uganda.

In: The Journey …
Editors: Robert Basaza et al.
ISBN: 978-1-53618-323-8

Chapter 2

ASSESSMENT OF THE FEASIBILITY OF SUBSIDIZING HEALTH INSURANCE FOR TARGET GROUPS IN UGANDA

Donald Shapard[1,*], Prossy K. Namyalo[2], Aggrey Kihombo[3] and Robert Basaza[4,5]
[1]Brandeis University, Waltham, MA, US
[2]Ndejje University, Faculty of Social Sceinces,Uganda
[3]Mzumbe University, Tanzania
[4]Gudie Incubation Centre, Kira Municipality, Uganda
[5]Uganda Christian University Mukono MPHL Program, Uganda

ABSTRACT

Using data from the literature, documents, and interviews with stakeholders, this study which was commissioned by USAID Uganda, examined the cost-effectiveness of reproductive health vouchers (RHVs) and subsidy of community-based health insurance to improve maternal outcomes in Uganda.

* Corresponding Author's E-mail: shepard@brandeis.edu.

According to World Health Organization, a service is considered highly cost effective if it can generate a disability adjusted life year (DALY) at a cost below the country's gross domestic product (GDP) per capita [1, 2]. The study found that both vouchers and community-based health insurance (CBHI) are highly cost-effective. At most likely costs of US$302 per DALY averted for vouchers and $309 for subsidy of CBHI. both interventions are highly cost-effective and virtually identical in their cost-effectiveness ratios. Both cost-effectiveness ratios are below US$510, Uganda's GDP per capita. On policy grounds, the subsidy of CBHI is more consistent with a broader policy supported by Uganda and other partner states in the East African community of expanding social health protection through enrolling the population in universal health insurance.

Insurance should also include outreach to encourage poor women to deliver at health facilities, transportation to and from health centers for deliveries, and incentives to health workers for increased volume and improved quality. In the neighboring country of Rwanda, with a health system like that of Uganda offering government, non-government, or faith-based health facilities, such incentives proved successful in improving use of primary care services. Insurance models that create sustainable incentives for providers to offer quality care have the potential to increase access through partnerships between care providers and member groups or CBHI plans. This chapter is an update from the original text presented to the Ugandan Health Sector in 2015.

ABBREVIATIONS

AL	Artemether-lumefatrine;
ANC	Antenatal care;
ASH	African Strategies for Health;
CBHI	Community-based health insurance: DALY: Disability adjusted life year;
DFID	Department for International Development (UK);
DHS	Demographic and Health Survey;
FP	Family planning;
GDP	Gross domestic product;
GOU	Government of Uganda;
HF	Health facility;
HMO	Health Maintenance Organization;

HP	HealthPartners;
ICER	Incremental cost-effectiveness ratio;
IML	International Medical Link;
IMR	Infant mortality rate;
IUD	Intra-uterine device;
KfW	German Development Bank;
KNBOS	Kenya National Bureau of Statistics;
LTM	Long-term method;
MDG	Millennium Development Goal;
MILO	Medical Insurance for Low Income;
MMR	Maternal mortality rate;
MoHCDGEM	Ministry of Health, Community Development, Gender, Elderly and Children;
MOU	Memorandum of Understanding;
MSI	Marie Stopes International;
MSU	Marie Stopes Uganda;
NHIS	National health insurance scheme;
OBA	Output-based aid;
OOP	Out-of-pocket;
P4H	Providing for Health;
P4P	Pay for performance;
PBIs	Performance-based incentives;
PMTCT	Prevention of mother to child transmission;
PNFPs	Private not-for-profits;
RBF	Results-based financing;
RHV	Reproductive Health Vouchers;
SHU	Save for Health Uganda;
SMGL	Saving Mothers Giving Lives;
THE	Total health expenditure;
UBOS	Uganda Bureau of Statistics;
UCBHFA	Uganda Community Based Health Financing Association;
UGX	Uganda shillings;
USAID	United States Agency for International Development;

VS	Voucher schemes;
WHO	World Health Organization;
WRA	Women of reproductive age;
YLD	Years lost from disability;
YLL	Years of life lost.

INTRODUCTION

Uganda and its development partners have implemented a number of financial approaches to improve access to health services, and particularly in the reproductive health services sector. Uganda's second health policy specifies that the sector shall establish overall adjusted health financing mechanisms based on pre-payment and financial risk pooling aiming at universal coverage and social health protection. These includes; national health insurance and other community health financing mechanisms [3]. There are over 24 community-based health insurance (CBHI) schemes, including six health cooperatives that are financially owned and managed by local stakeholders in Southwestern Uganda. The schemes started as a result of USAID-funded support by Health Partners (HP).

The country's Out-of-Pocket Expenditure (OOP), as a Proportion of Total Health Expenditure (THE) stands at 42% [4] and 28% of Ugandan households experience catastrophic health expenditures [5]. Recognizing that rising OOP puts poor and limited-income populations at risk of incurring catastrophic health expenditures, the government abolished user fees in 2001. However, evidence suggests that increased private expenditure on drugs and hospital/clinic fees (including informal payments at public facilities) offsets the impact of the abolition of user fees.

The absence of adequate risk-pooling arrangements is an obstacle to ensuring individuals' greater access to needed health care and leaves them at risk of catastrophic OOP payments in the event of illness. The population with private or community health insurance is negligible in Uganda (about 2%). Uganda also lacks a national health insurance scheme (NHIS), although it is currently in the policy dialogue. The Providing for Health

(P4H) Network (World Health Organization, WHO, World Bank, etc.) is currently supporting the Government of Uganda (GOU) to develop the NHIS. While both private, commercial and community health insurance schemes are expected to be incorporated into the NHIS, as was done in other countries, any meaningful rollout is considered unlikely in the medium term. From 2008-2011, KfW (German Development Bank) and the World Bank funded a "healthy baby" safe delivery voucher which rolled out a pilot project in private health insurance providers in Western Uganda. The project was implemented by Marie Stopes International and targeted women of reproductive age (WRA) from the bottom two quintiles of the consumption distribution. However, person-level means testing was not followed everywhere. In some locations, all pregnant women from the targeted geographical areas were considered eligible [6, 7]. Eligible pregnant women could purchase a voucher for a subsidized fee (3,000 UGX, or roughly $1.40 USD) from an accredited voucher service provider, which covered four antenatal care visits, delivery care, referral and treatment of eventual complications, and a postnatal care visit. The providers were either Private for Profit (PFP) or Private Not-for-Profit (PNFP) facilities and offered basic and comprehensive emergency obstetric care depending on their capacity. In 2010, over forty thousand (41,487) vouchers were sold and 28,182 (68%) redeemed for the delivery portion [8]. As of June 2011, over 50,000 Healthy Baby vouchers had been sold and 40,000 redeemed for the delivery portion of the service package [9].

The United States Agency for International Development and the UK's Department for International Development (DFID) are currently funding Marie Stopes Uganda (MSU) to implement a nationwide Long Term Method (LTM) Family Planning (FP) voucher program. From 2012 to 2013, USAID funded a safe delivery voucher program in the Saving Mothers Giving Lives (SMGL) districts in Western Uganda. A consortium of donors, including USAID, has nationwide scale up of the healthy baby voucher. This culminated into the USAID/Uganda Voucher Plus Activity, a five-year (2016-2021) USAID-funded results based financing mechanism implemented by Abt Associates, in partnership with Communication for Development Foundation Uganda (CDFU), Price Waterhouse Coopers

(PwC) and BDO-East Africa. The Activity is designed to increase access to quality obstetric, newborn, and postpartum family planning services to poor women through the private sector in 33 districts in Northern and Eastern Uganda so as to contribute to the reduction of maternal and newborn mortality and morbidity.

Uganda's Community-Based Health Insurance (CBHI) schemes are coordinated by the umbrella organization called Uganda Community Based Health Financing Association (UCBHFA). Most of the current schemes are hospital-managed and are small in terms of population coverage. Most of the participating service providers are PNFP organizations which partly subsidize the costs of CBHI clients through ongoing donor subsidies such as free medicines. Experience has shown that when donors subsidize CBHI, the uptake increases dramatically and falls again when the subsidy is withdrawn [10]. The government declaration of "free" health care services, and widespread lack of understanding of the concept of insurance, further jeopardizes the scale-up of CBHI because beneficiaries are expected to pay premiums.

Remarkably, donors perceive that, vouchers are able to support quick improvements in reproductive health. Nevertheless, supporting the expansion of CBHI could contribute to a longer-term goal of universal coverage for health care. The subsidized CBHI might eventually form part of an NHIS-type system (as supported by the Global Fund for AIDS, Tuberculosis, and Malaria in Rwanda and USAID in Ethiopia). This may be more cost-effective (measured by unit cost of deaths averted or reduced morbidity) than support to vertical voucher programs. A case in point is where a private health provider in the HP-supported CBHI program charges UGX 20,000 per person per year for an expanded package of services (including Long Term Methods (LTM) and safe deliveries), while the MSU LTM voucher reimbursement for a provider works out to about UGX 20,000 for an intra-uterine device (IUD) procedure alone. (Note: in July 2014, the exchange rate was 2568 UGX per US dollar). Similarly, the administrative overhead of managing a program offering an expanded package of services may be more cost-effective than multiple vertical programs, especially if a capitation model is used with providers, incentivized to reduce fraud and waste. When high penetration is achieved in a CBHI scheme, the costs of services are considerably reduced due to economies of scale. The provider incentives further minimizes financial costs and increases efficient use of resources. The economies of scale available to health providers by donors that subsidizes the target group of clients results in the cost of services being reduced so that CBHI's are affordable to more people. Kampala International University and Teaching Hospital, trained by HealthPartners, enrolled health cooperative members in tiered benefit packages with plans to use surpluses from higher tiers to offer subsidized care to vulnerable populations.

The evidence suggests that reaching the Millennium Development Goal (MDG) 5 of reducing maternal mortality rate (MMR) by 75% by 2015 was quite challenging for most, if not all, developing countries [11]. In Uganda, while remarkable success was achieved in reducing MMR from 600 in 1990 to 300 in 2010, a decrease of 47% in that time period [12, 13, 14] attaining a reduction of 75% by 2015 would mean lowering this rate further to 131 [15]. Achieving this result within a one-year period would require a greater rate of reduction than currently exists. In providing services for reproductive health, both vouchers and CBHI fund key services. About 18.1% of deaths of women aged 15-49 years are maternal [15]. Health care during pregnancy is applauded for saving the lives of women [16] as most maternal deaths can be prevented with access to quality and skilled antenatal care (ANC), appropriate facilities for deliveries, postnatal care [17], and access to family planning [18]. However, access to maternal health care has remained persistently low in most resource-constrained countries, especially affecting women in low-income quintiles [19, 20]. This has been a major limiting factor in reducing the MMR. The Uganda Bureau of Statistics indicated access to maternal care was at 60% of the number of pregnant women who made four or more ANC visits during their pregnancy. It showed that 74% of the births were assisted by a skilled health providers and barely 73% of the births were delivered at health facilities. Further, 54% of women received postnatal care in their first 2 days after delivery [21].

Barriers to women's access to maternal services have ranged from transport costs, high service fees at health facilities, and long distances to health service points. Other barriers include, insufficient supplies of drugs and equipment at the health facilities, poor provider training and treatment with patients, among other challenges [22, 23, 24]. Increasing women's access to maternal services is an important strategy in addressing MMR, and one way of reaching that goal is by improving health care financing through the budget, yet the budget system is seen to have some flaws. The economic capacity of Uganda is weak to sufficiently and equitably finance its health care systems. Only seven percent of the government budget is provided for health, which is far less than 15% committed by African Heads of State in Abuja, Nigeria [25, 26].

The second concern about the current financing system is its orientation of being more of a supply-side strategy, which is criticized for distributing money to government agencies without regard to achieving allocative efficiency [19]. The system is also criticized for lack of incentives to providers to increase their performance to attract clients to their services (ibid). The supply-side approach ignores the demand-side. Clients' access to health care is not only barred by shortages of supplies in health facilities but also by other factors such as distance, price of health commodities, and transport fare among other things. These are factors that any good financing mechanism should take into consideration (ibid). As a result of the shortcomings in the supply-side financing, some countries and health partners have suggested demand-side financing, starting with community-based health insurance schemes [27, 28]. However, enrollment in most of these schemes has generally remained low. The pattern elucidates, 3% for some schemes in Nigeria (in 2009), 1.4% in Guinea (in 2006), 1% in Kenya [29], and 2% in Uganda [30]. Enrollment in Uganda ranges from 5%-10% in places where the schemes are located. Moreover, the schemes are characterized by income and distance inequalities for membership and access [31, 28].

Voucher coverage can be higher than that of CBHI. Vouchers paid for 38% of deliveries of poor women in targeted districts. While vouchers appear to create a parallel mechanism for reimbursing reproductive health services, they can also be seen as a mechanism to promote universal health care through their ability to synchronize services, increase equity by focusing subsidy on the poor, expanding the package of care, and improving quality of care [8, 32]. Since both voucher and CBHI have common goals of increasing access to reproductive health services by WRA, it is necessary to know where to invest more. This analysis of the options permits comparison between subsidized health insurance and vouchers and scrutinizes other policies, such as conditional cash transfers and other demand-side financing. For example, in Rwanda under "community resource-based financing," pregnant women receive items for their babies if they deliver at a health facility instead of delivering at home. To address these needs, USAID/Uganda requested this study from the African Strategies for Health (ASH) project to assess cost-effectiveness and policy options when comparing community-based health insurance to voucher schemes in Uganda.

METHODS

Conceptual Frameworks

The ideal data for quantitative assessments of subsidized CBHI and vouchers would be a controlled design with comparison groups, preferably randomized. If available, such study would compare rates of use of a service and outcomes under a subsidized CBHI, with vouchers, or neither. Unfortunately, no such data were found in Uganda. The strongest design possible with available data was a combination of difference-in-difference analyses and multi-variable regression. The former technique requires pre- and post-intervention data on recipients, and data on a comparable control population before and after the intervention period. This design allows the evaluator to check on the comparability between intervention and control groups and to use the baseline value for each group to control for any remaining differences. Multi-variable regression allowed estimation of the effect of increasing enrollment in CBHI in a geographical area on the rate of institutional deliveries in that area.

Data Collection

The study team used three data and information gathering methods during the assessment: desk reviews, key informant interviews, and observations. First, the team reviewed key historical data and other literature. These documents included the benefit packages of key CBHI and voucher schemes listing services covered, price lists, grant and contract agreements, budgets, technical and financial reports. Others were strategy and policy documents, tools, publications, and any other relevant materials documenting the implementation process, cost, results and effects. USAID/Uganda's assistance was sought to identify some of these materials.

Second, the study team conducted in-depth interviews with key informants. The study team developed an interview guide that included opinions and data about the functioning of the program, the reasons for the design, and the use of services and costs. The researchers enlisted help from USAID to identify key informants. The key informants included scheme operators, donors supporting these programs, commercial insurers, government policy makers, service providers, and consumers.

Finally, using direct field observations, the study team made visits to sites where CBHI and voucher schemes were being implemented. These were sites in Bushenyi and Mbarara Districts in Western Uganda alongside Health Membership Organizations (HMOs) and other plans in Kampala. With closed panels of physicians, HMOs in Uganda resemble Health Maintenance Organizations in the US. Most CBHI schemes and previous voucher programs were mainly based in Western Uganda.

Cost Analysis

The cost analysis examined costs to the sponsoring organization and to the health system overall. The latter included costs paid by households and government. For patient-level costs, the cost analysis used the following equation for each type of service:

Total cost = Unit cost x quantity

Quantity represents the number of services a person receives during the time period under study (a pregnancy or a year). For a one-time service, such as a delivery, the quantity is the percentage of persons who receive the service. The types of services are those paid by CBHI or the voucher. If the effectiveness or unit cost of a service varies by setting, then each setting constitutes a separate type of service. In theory, pre-natal visits could be listed as a type of service. However, these services are free in government clinics. Also, they do not require many supplies or equipment and because government clinics are generally more numerous, they likely entail less travel time. The resulting services are:

- Program administration
- Paid transport to referral
- Homebirth and public delivery
- Private delivery, non-output-based aid (OBA) and Private delivery, OBA

In addition to patient-level costs, organizational-level costs are tallied (e.g., technical assistance for policy and guideline development and revisions, trainings, facilities, consumer enrollment, communication and marketing, staff time for operations, demand-side and patient costs). Finally, intangible inputs (e.g., political will, operational efficiencies, and other costs that cannot be easily measured in terms of dollars) were noted and described.

Evaluation of Outcomes

Based on the literature review, the impact of CBHI was evaluated in Rwanda through a multi-variable regression analysis as part of a study of the impact of HIV/AIDS services in health care delivery [33]. The CBHI, operationalized as mutuelle coverage (mutuelleco, the percentage of the catchment population enrolled in CBHI) was included as one of the control variables. The units of analysis were 52 rural health centers in Rwanda. Secondary analyses examined impacts on primary health care services [34] and on maternal health services [35]. The key impact measure for the latter was the natural logarithm of the "delivery rate", namely the percentage of deliveries in the health center's catchment area that occurred at the facility, where the alternative was a home-based delivery. These analyses used the logarithmic transformation because the volume of services could vary substantially, and different kinds of services could be analyzed in a parallel way. The major service outcomes for vouchers came from Alfonso et al. and Mazzilli [9, 24].

The impact on health outcomes was based on the risks and benefits of alternative types of services derived from Uganda-specific data from Alfonso et al. and Mazzilli [9, 24]. These were expressed as the mortality and morbidity rates for a cohort of a specified size, e.g., 25,000 women. In addition, the evaluation considers intangible effects (e.g., institutional capacity, consumer morale, and motivation). The analysis allowed us to evaluate whether the incremental effects of scheme implementation were worth the costs.

Qualitative Analysis

Qualitative data which was obtained from the site observations and interviews was analyzed using a separate approach to elucidate emergent themes, contextual factors, and trends. This information and the documents obtained provided information on several voucher schemes in Uganda.

Key Outcomes

Both vouchers and subsidized CBHI are intended to increase access to a quality delivery at a health facility by a pregnant woman, as well as other services. The facility should be clean, appropriately equipped, staffed by trained personnel, and backed up by emergency transport and referral plans

Review of literature of the voucher programs highlight the importance of the schemes with three key outcome areas: i) target of specific groups or programs, ii) promotion of utilization, and iii) advancement of quality [20]. To date, evidence on targeting suggests that voucher programs tended to serve the poorer population more than those who were richer [38]. For example, when a voucher program that targeted low-income people was introduced in Uganda, fewer women reported lack of money as the reason barring them to seek treatment [38].

Table 2. Voucher system and maternal utilization in selected countries

Country	Health indicator	Before or Control Group	After or Treatment Group
Bangladesh	Used at least 3 ANC	33.6%	54.8%
	Deliveries attended by skilled provider	27.1%	63.7%
	Health facility-based deliveries	18.7%	37.5%
	C-Section	9.1%	10.4%
Cambodia	Health facility-based deliveries	16.4%	44.0%
India	Home deliveries	21.0%	0.4%
	Deliveries at private health facility	77.0%	97.0%
Kenya	Health facility-based deliveries	64.7%	71.9%
Uganda	Home deliveries	30.0%	17.0%

Source: Bellows et al. (2013).

Impact of Vouchers on Quality

Concerning the impact of vouchers on quality, it was found that most evaluated projects had positive impact, as revenues from the vouchers were used to improve health facility infrastructure, hire more medical staff, acquire new equipment, and replenish supplies and stocks [38].

Cost and Effectiveness of Vouchers in Uganda

The study by Alfonso provides the most thorough analysis on vouchers in Uganda. Under usual care in Uganda, as of 2011, the rate of health facility

(HF)-based deliveries in rural areas was 54% of all deliveries [15]. In addition, 94% of all pregnant women have at least one ANC visit [15]. The overall institutional delivery coverage for the baseline study was 58.9% [24]. The primary source of data for estimating the impact of vouchers is the previously cited cost-effectiveness study in Uganda [24]. This study, involving both the private and public health facilities modeled a voucher program which covered costs of delivery and provision of round trip transportation using private sector workers' bicycles or motorcycles.

The unit costs for services are noted as: transport reimbursement which was \$1.8 - US\$4.5 (2009 dollars) per woman receiving transport for delivery. Health facility services' reimbursement ranged from US\$2.87 - US\$5.75. The nominal payment to a facility for a C-Section was US\$27 - \$59. Private HFs received 100% of the voucher's nominal reimbursement value. Public HFs received at most 75% of the standard reimbursement for the value [24]. Unpublished data showed that during 2008-2010, the economic cost of delivery in public health facilities in Uganda was US\$17.62 [9, 24]. In a study in Masaka, Uganda during a period of cost sharing by Levin et al. (2000), the cost of delivery at public HFs was found to be US\$3.33 while at private HFs it was US\$18.79 [24]. Alfonso et al. drew on cost data from Mazzilli and from Levin et al. (2000), which estimated US\$ 17.62 for public and US\$ 18.79 for private HF delivery costs. These HF costs excluded OOP payments made by patients; these amounted to US\$10.68 according to Bellows and Hamilton in Alfonso et al. The discount rate for the life years saved was 3% [9, 24, 39].

Table 3 lists the input parameters from the voucher program. Table 4 shows the unadjusted outputs—deliveries at HFs participating in the voucher program. These results found that the rate of deliveries for women at participating HFs was nearly twice (74%) those without vouchers (36%). Regression results indicated that the demand for deliveries at health facilities enrolled in the program rose by 52.3 percentage points after the scheme was introduced. However, much of this change was a transfer from deliveries that would have taken place elsewhere. After reviewing facility registers and adjusting conservatively for missing data, Alfonso and colleagues estimated that facility-based deliveries increased by 9.4 percentage points. Alfonso et al. projected the impact of applying the voucher program to a hypothetical population of 1 million persons. The increase in facility-based deliveries would lead to 20 lives saved.

Table 3. Model parameters and assumptions for the voucher program

Label	Parameter	Value	Low	Hig	Source
	Decision tree probabilities				
A	Institutional delivery if voucher scheme	0.68	0.57	0.79	MUSPH (2009)
B	Institutional delivery if status quo	0.59	0.51	0.65	MUSPH (2009); UBOS & ICF (20102)
C	% of deliveries at public HF (vs. Home)	58%	41%	58%	
D	Referral proportion	0.9%			Calculated
	Costs				
E	Average program costs per				
	Delivery (private or public)	$19.65	$19.65	$24.63	
	Public HF referral	$32.16	$25.63	$32.16	
	Private HF referral	$59.73	$51.16	$59.73	
F	HF costs for				
	Public delivery	$17.62	$3.33	$18.77	Mazzilli (2011); Levin et al. (2000)
	Public referral	$65.65	$65.65	$89.71	Mazzilli (2011); Levin et al. (2000)
	Public subsidy to private HF per delivery	$4.70	$3.32	$12.53	Levin et al. (2000)
	Public subsidy to private HF per referral	$26.53	$18.73	$70.75	Levin et al. (2000)
	Private delivery	$18.79			Levin et al. (2000)
	Private referral	$106.13			Levin et al. (2000)
G	OOP costs for				
	Delivery & referral (private or public HF)	$10.68	$3.27	$22.44	Bellows and Hamilton (2009)
	HF round trip transportation	$4.60	$3.73	$6.14	
	Care giver lost gross domestic product/day	$1.33			
H	HF capital cost estimate per delivery	$2.68			Mazzilli (2011)
I	LiST parameters				
	Hypothetical population cohort	1,000,000			
	National population (1000s)	33,425			UN (2011)
	Rural total fertility	6.7	3.8	6.7	Kakande (2011) unpublished
	National total fertility	6.2	3.8	6.2	Kakande (2011) unpublished
	Rural HIV prevalence	5.7	5.3	5.9	Uganda Ministry of Health (2006)
	National HIV prevalence	6.4	5.3	6.4	Uganda Ministry of Health (2006)
	TT Tetanus toxoid vaccination	66%			
	IPTp	55%			
	Clean birth practices	62%			

Source: Alfonso et al. (2013).

Table 4. Impact of vouchers on deliveries: Percentage of women delivering at a health facility by control and intervention group

Time period	Control	Intervention
Before	30%	16%
After	36%	74%
Improvement	6%	58%
Net impact		52%

Source: Alfonso et al. (2013).

These are equivalent to 1356 DALYs averted, the sum of 477 years of life lost (YLLs) and 879 years of life with disability (YLDs). The incremental cost-effectiveness ratio (ICER) per DALYs averted was US$ 302/DALY and per death averted was US$ 20,756 [24].

DALY as It Applies to CBHI

It is important to examine the DALY calculation so that it can be done in a parallel way for evaluating the impact of CBHI. The study estimates that a 9.4 percentage point increase in attended deliveries would yield a total of 20 lives saved in the impact year. These 20 lives saved are equivalent to 1356 DALYs averted [24]. For rural Uganda as a whole, the crude birth rate in 2011 was 42.1 per 1000 population [15]. The hypothetical population of 1,000,000 persons would have 42,100 births per year. The share of births delivered at a HF for women in the poorest wealth quintile was 42.2%. Therefore, a 9.4 percentage point increase in attended deliveries in the hypothetical population would increase the number of HF births by 3,958 (i.e., 42,100 x 9.4%). One DALY is gained for each 2.94 additional HF deliveries. These DALYs are, presumably, the combination of lower maternal mortality, maternal morbidity (e.g., obstetrical fistula and malaria), and infant morbidity and mortality. Since CBHI also operates through facility-based service delivery and targets similar health facility services, it is useful to apply the same parameters.

Projected Impact of CBHI

Enrollment in health insurance is relatively low in Uganda. In 2011, only 1.2% of women and 1.8% of men were enrolled in any health insurance. Among those in the poorest wealth quintile, only 0.2% of women and 1.1% of men were enrolled [15]. As a result, existing data for estimating the utilization under health insurance in Uganda are limited. The data, however, is useful for estimating costs and providing descriptive information on utilization. Three examples of CBHI in Uganda are presented.

Medical Insurance for Low Income

In 2014, the company International Medical Link (IML) initiated a scheme called Medical Insurance for Low Income (MILO). For residents of rural areas, the monthly premium is UGX 7,000 (US$ 2.50) or US $30 per year. The product is fully licensed by the Insurance Regulatory Authority of Uganda. This scheme covers children and adults without regard to pregnancy status. The scheme operates in Western Uganda (Mbarara), Central (Kampala), and Northern Uganda (Gulu). As of July 21, 2014, the scheme had been operating about 5 months. It had 351 subscribed members (184 males and 167 females). Of the female members, 98 were women of reproductive age (WRA between 15-49 years of age). They represented 28% of the subscribers. For rural Uganda overall, WRA represented 19.7% of the population [15]. The company indicated that teachers (a professional group) and boda-boda (motorcycle) transporters, fishermen, and others with some disposable income were targeted. The difference in the share of the population comprised by WRA likely reflects the fact that children and/or elders were under-represented among the subscribers. The quality of data from MILO is reinforced by the crude birth rate among subscribers of 28.5 per 1000 population (5 births in 175.2 person years). The rate for rural Uganda, a less educated population, was 42.5 [15].

Save for Health Uganda

Save for Health Uganda (SHU) offers a variety of prepayment products including a mix of credit-based and insurance-based products for healthcare. Save for Health Uganda has an insurance or prepayment product specifically targeting pregnant women [40]. Its reproductive health program operates primarily around Sheema district health facilities in Western Uganda. While full documentation is not available, it appears that the premium for a pregnant woman is the same as that for the general population, which is UGX 20,000 (about US $8.00) per year. Since a pregnant woman would be expected to consume more services, the scheme likely loses money on these enrollees. However, the financial data shows that donor contributions (with Bread for the World being the largest), are an important part of the organization's operations. A particularly noteworthy feature about this program is the coverage of boda-boda (motorcycle) transporters to bring pregnant women to and from contracted health care facilities. The scheme had contracts with 20 such transport operators in 2013. Another noteworthy feature of SHU is that it has a union of schemes that provides reinsurance.

The Save for Health Uganda product reported having 33,369 beneficiaries in 2013 and an operating budget of US $622,450. This works out to a cost of $18.65 per beneficiary. The documentation was not very complete, but it is likely that this amount is just the management cost. The report did not indicate the percentage of beneficiaries who enrolled for the entire year (fees are collected quarterly, and beneficiaries can drop after one or two quarters), but the cost per person year would be higher. To illustrate, if the turnover was 33% (very likely), then 67% of beneficiaries would each contribute 1.0 person year, while 33% would contribute 0.5 person years each. Then the person years per beneficiary would be 0.83 and the management cost per beneficiary year would be $22.41. Therefore, the total cost per person insured would be $30 ($22.41 +$8). Furthermore, SHU operates a variety of programs, so the cost per beneficiary does not apply exclusively to CBHI. Nevertheless, the cost per beneficiary-year is comparable to the annual rural premium of MILO. Unlike vouchers, the scheme also covered immunizations and curative services. SHU reported that malaria was by far the single most frequent illness. With 1,550 malarial illnesses treated in the year, the rate was about 0.05 per beneficiary year. Save for Health Uganda reported that the utilization of obstetrics services in the Sheema district schemes was far better than the district and national utilization levels. The ANC 4 completion rate was 72%; the rate of institutional delivery was 75.1% and the rate of attendance at post-natal care was 11.6%. While both MILO and SHU offer CBHI to pregnant women, pregnant women have higher utilization of services than average members, so pregnant women's premiums are, in effect, subsidized by those other members.

Health Cooperatives

Health care cooperatives (coops) are associations of health care providers. The coops offer benefit packages to groups who share risk by paying quarterly premiums directly to the provider. This arrangement keeps administrative costs low and creates a partnership between health facilities and the communities they serve. Providers manage member relations through annually renewed Memorandums of Understanding (MOUs). Providers and coop members elect a board of directors to make leadership decisions to sustain benefits for all coop stakeholders.

In Uganda, USAID funding has been used to build the capacity of coop stakeholders while they establish locally sustainable systems. While the health coop model existed for many years, USAID increased investments in Uganda in 2011, which, according to data from USAID Uganda, resulted in 31,181 health coop members by June 2014. As of 2014, two of six health coops have opened bank accounts where they deposit annual membership fees and 10% of providers' annual surpluses from coop partnerships. Coop funds are used by boards to hold annual general meetings and quarterly board meetings.

Health coops improve provider quality because member groups sign MOUs with the provider of their choice. The HP has trained health coop stakeholders to elect quality care committees who work with their health facilities to conduct participatory provider quality assessments. During the last steps of this process, health coop members and care providers develop action plans together and then meet six months later so they can hold each other accountable to meet the quality standards they set.

Modeled Impact of CBHI on Delivery Rates in Uganda

We did not find any data from Uganda that would show the impact of CBHI on utilization of deliveries. In that absence, we used analyses from Uganda's neighbor, Rwanda. As the two countries have a mixed health system that combine public and PNFP facilities. Uganda and Rwanda also have almost a similar 2013 per capita gross national income in purchasing power parity ($1370 for Uganda, $1430 for Rwanda), Rwanda's experience should be informative for Uganda [41]. The multi-variable regression analysis by in the Rwandan context, found that a 1% increase in the health insurance enrollment rate of the entire population raises the delivery rate by 0.9% of its initial value [35]. This conclusion was based on the finding that the regression coefficient of health insurance coverage (termed mutuelle coverage (mutuelleco)) on the natural logarithm of the delivery rate was 0.009 and was highly significant ($p<.001$). The logarithm was used to adjust for extreme variability in delivery rates. We applied this relationship to rural Uganda, where the HF delivery rate was 42.2%. If 10% of the population were covered under CBHI and used their insurance, then the HF delivery rate would increase by 4.2 percentage points to 46.4%. In 1,000 pregnant women, the increase of 4.2 percentage points corresponds to 42 additional HF deliveries. Using the relationship from Alfonso et al. that 2.94 deliveries correspond to one DALY, the added coverage would correspond to 14.29 DALYs gained through insurance coverage of maternity services [24].

CBHI's Impact on Service Utilization for Malaria

A benefit of subsidized CBHI is its contribution to averting other causes of mortality for WRA. This could help with malaria, pneumonia, and other risks. Analysis of the data set also used by showed that CBHI led to significant increases in the use of three services at health centers to derive the resulting gain in DALYs [34, 35]. We focused on malaria, as the data from SHU showed it to be the predominant cause of ambulatory visits. Data from the Institute of Health Metrics and Evaluation (2014) showed that malaria caused 2,399,530 DALYs in 2010. In that year, the population of Uganda was 33,425,000. On that basis, our model population of 1,000 people would lose 71.8 DALYs. A randomized trial in Uganda found that the most effective treatment for malaria (artemether-lumefatrine, AL) had a failure rate of only 6.7% of episodes, compared to an average rate of 21.8% for the two comparative treatments [42]. Thus, the correct treatment would reduce the failure rate by 69% (i.e., 100% - 6.7%/21.8%). Yet, an evaluation of Uganda's health system found that 40% of outpatient consultations failed to receive the recommended treatment (AL) for malaria [43]. A major factor was the lack of the appropriate dosage of the AL treatment. We projected, and experience from Rwanda which largely confirms that the funding and community oversight through CBHI could largely erase such deficits. Combining these factors, the hypothesized 10% increase in CBHI would avert 5.6 DALYs from malarial illness in pregnant women. If a woman received insurance to cover both maternity and malaria-related services, she would avert 19.88 (14.28+5.6) DALYs. This approximation is conservative, in that it does not project the benefits of insurance coverage on other services that address the other leading causes of mortality and morbidity in WRA, such as other infections.

If insurance were offered as a household package to the average household size of five persons [21] including the pregnant women, the benefits would be five times 5.6 DALYs (from general insurance) plus 14.28 DALYs (from coverage for pregnancy-related services). Thus, the total impact would be 42.3 DALYs averted.

Cost-Effectiveness of CBHI

To calculate the cost-effectiveness of subsidizing CBHI, we need to project the cost of subsidizing CBHI for poor, pregnant women. We present the most favorable and most likely estimates. The most favorable assumption is that CBHI is offered to pregnant women at the premium for the general population. The most likely estimate is that the premium for insuring a poor pregnant woman would be based on the actuarial cost of the services received. It is useful to explain the most favorable assumption. We noted earlier that the MILO and SHU cost of insurance is about $30 per person per year. CBHI is based on the principle of risk sharing whereby healthy subscribers support those who are sick or otherwise need services. The initial experience of MILO is consistent with this assumption. As long as the birth rate among MILO subscribers is comparable to the Ugandan crude birth rate (42.4 births per 1000 population), it is likely that the plan will remain financially sound. On the other hand, if donors offered to subsidize the prevailing cost of insurance only for poor WRA enrolled, the birth rate would be 1000 per 1000 population—24 times the current rate, and the need for services would be similarly higher. A massive increase in the number of general population (non-WRA) clients would be needed to subsidize the cost of this additional service to WRA—such as by enrolling entire families. In the prevailing environment, such an organic increase in general population clients is very unlikely. The most likely scenario assumption is that some subsidy, a higher premium, or a cross-subsidy from other insured beneficiaries would be needed to support the added services required to support an increase in poor WRA enrollment.

We estimated the additional cost of covering a pregnant woman, as compared to a member of the general population, based on the following considerations. Based on [24], we estimated the cost of a normal delivery (public or private facility) at $19.65, and a private referral (e.g., for a C-section) at $106.13. We assumed the rate of C-section would be that of women in Uganda who are in the highest wealth quintile, 12.6% [15]. This assumption was based on the findings from site visits to HMOs in Kampala that their enrollees were mostly upper middle-class women who preferred the convenience of a known schedule. A normal delivery thus had a probability of 87.4% (i.e., 100.0% - 12.6%). This gave a gross cost for a delivery of $30.55. However, the premium already covers the average probability of 4.21% of a pregnancy, for an expected cost of $1.29. Thus, the additional pregnancy cost was $29.26. The most likely cost for one year for insurance for a pregnant woman would be $59.26. Our projections for insurance were based on 10% coverage for the hypothetical population of 1000 persons. These correspond to $3,000 for the most favorable, and $5,926 for the most likely. As noted, the health gains are 19.88 DALYs. These give cost effectiveness ratios of $221 (most favorable), and $298 (most likely).

Cost-Effectiveness Comparison

The preceding analysis finds $302 per DALY as the best estimate for the voucher. For subsidized CBHI, our most favorable assumption leads to $150 per DALY. Our most likely estimate is $298 per DALY.

DISCUSSION

This analysis has found that both community-based health insurance (CBHI) and vouchers have proved useful in Uganda and elsewhere in contributing to improved access and quality of health services. The improvement in access works in four ways: (1) little or no out-of-pocket charges for facility-based services both for normal and complicated deliveries, (2) subsidy for transport services for delivery and for transfer from a primary facility to a hospital for emergency obstetric services, (3) in some cases, advocacy by the transport operator, who may encourage the pregnant woman to go to a health facility, and (4) marketing of the voucher to the poor.

The improvement in quality occurs through (1) deliveries at facilities operated by non-governmental organizations (NGOs) and private for-profit providers which are generally considered to be of higher quality than government facilities, and (2) specific quality criteria managed by the voucher management agency, which include adequate staffing, adequate training, and presence of key supplies and working equipment, including access to a working ambulance for emergency transfers. Data limitations have created uncertainties around the benefits of each of these improvements.

Many of the same private health facilities (especially PNFPs) participated in both the Healthy Baby voucher program, as well as in CBHI schemes, and will likely do so again when the multi-donor safe delivery voucher program re-starts. This will constitute a hidden subsidy for CBHI. However, even without a voucher program in place, donors (especially USAID and DFID) routinely provide free quality improvement advice and free essential medicines to PNFPs. This suggests that in the absence of a voucher program, the incremental cost of increasing quality of safe delivery services at PNFPs to match those at private for profit might be marginal. A benefit of subsidized CBHI is its contribution to averting other causes of mortality for WRA. This could help with malaria, pneumonia, and other risks.

An additional factor to consider in comparing the cost-effectiveness of vouchers and CBHI is whether and how much they improve uptake of family planning services. In bringing WRA in contact with the health system, where the women see posters, interact with health professionals, and talk with other clients, both interventions should contribute to higher uptake. The impact should be greater for CBHI, however, because it covers services longer after delivery when a woman's fertility returns. Thus, CBHI should have a greater impact on the number of maternal deaths (because there are fewer pregnancies), and on MMR because there are fewer high-risk pregnancies (e.g., those in very young women). The Government of Uganda and its development partners' goal is to increase use of modern family planning, as evidenced by the existence of voucher programs for family planning. We are not aware of data, however, which quantify the contribution of CBHI to increased use of family planning and improved maternal health in the Ugandan context although studies elsewhere have found mixed results [44].

Administrative Cost of Vouchers Compared with CBHI Administrative Costs

We do compare the administrative cost per person covered in subsidized CBHI compared to vouchers. Available data showed relatively similar costs per person covered in several programs: $22 for SHU provided CBHI, $19.65 for vouchers in the Alfonso et al. study, and $30 for the Healthy Baby Voucher Program. The USAID SHOPS/SMGL voucher program, implemented quickly as an emergency effort, showed higher costs of $91.48 per person. Subsidized CBHI relies more on local administration, whereas vouchers in Uganda and some other countries receive support from international organizations. As international involvement and management in vouchers is reduced, the administrative costs per person are likely to fall over time. However, the risk of insolvency from poor management could also increase. If in addition to safe delivery vouchers, the administrative cost of USAID's other voucher program, the Long-Term Methods (LTM) is considered ($52 per person covered according to project budgets from USAID Uganda, plus often other support to the sponsoring PNFP providers). It is very likely that the total administrative cost borne by USAID for supporting two separate voucher programs would significantly exceed that to support a subsidized CBHI program. This would be particularly true if the CBHI program were focused on PNFP service providers, as these already receive significant assistance (quality improvement, supplies, and training) from other USAID service delivery support programs. As such, the administrative costs per person of both vouchers and subsidized CBHI are likely to fall over time.

Challenges and Administrative Needs Associated with CBHI

Subsidized CBHI requires refinement of several administrative mechanisms. The first is regulation. Regulation is intended to ensure that insurers remain solvent and meet contractual obligations to cover beneficiaries and pay providers as promised. This is particularly the case if referral services owing to the fact that complications are covered on a fee-for-service basis. Uganda has an insurance regulatory mechanism that can provide oversight, but donors could also play a key role in guaranteeing financial solvency, perhaps through reinsurance. Frequent reporting, maintaining up-to-date financial records, and adjusting premiums and benefits can minimize such risks.

Another challenge is targeting of subsidies. Currently, some vouchers involve targeting at a household level (based on assets owned and other indicators), while others target geographically (specified sectors). Rwanda is beginning to address household-level targeting through differential premiums for community-based health insurance. The premiums are based on the classification of households in six economic strata from destitute to very rich under a system termed "ubudehe" based on their members' employment and ownership of land, livestock and other assets as recorded in administrative records of local government. Likely, a combination of strategies is necessary. In a few areas, such as those affected by famine, it might be safe to assume that all households are poor and geographical targeting is sufficient. In most places, however, household-level targeting will be needed. Tools used to assess eligibility in voucher programs need to be adapted to CBHI, staff need to be trained, and monitoring mechanisms need to be established to ensure that eligible households get included, but ineligible households do not receive subsidies inappropriately.

Management is another need. Both community-based and provider-based organizations, such as health coops, form viable bases. However, capacity building is needed to ensure that the organization is competent and remains honest. A CBHI management agency is needed for monitoring, reinsurance, and, targeting. Currently, USAID's Health Partners' Health Cooperatives project plays this role and through its MAMA cooperative, it is focused on WRA. It may be useful to link it with local government, where data for household-level targeting may already be available, or with the management of vouchers for reproductive health or family planning.

Data Limitations

While we believe the conceptual model underlying this study is robust, several limitations in the data must be acknowledged. Neither vouchers nor CBHI have been evaluated in the context of controlled trials. Observational data by Alfonso and Bellows [19, 24] about the net impact of vouchers on HF delivery rates attempt to control for confounding influences, but they are based on limited geographical areas and unequal changes between control and intervention areas in the health system or economy during the study period. This could confound the findings. The impact on health insurance is primarily based on one scheme (MILO) and statistical creation of a control group from the published Uganda DHS survey. Persons enrolling in health insurance may be more health conscious or differ in other ways that cannot be controlled for with available data. Finally, data are limited for estimating the cost of insurance specifically for pregnant women, who are known to need medical services, compared to a product for the general population or even WRA, who on average, have less health needs. Ongoing monitoring of whatever policies are implemented will provide data to test, and potentially overcome, these limitations.

Uganda has some additional experience with CBHI with Microcare, Kampala International University and Teaching Hospital and Comboni Hospital and with vouchers at Kantel, Kamuli and Pallisa Districts [24], and a World Bank-funded scheme which begun in 2015. If sufficient data from these settings become available, they could inform future cost-effectiveness analysis.

Conclusion and Recommendations

The considerations led to the following conclusions and recommendations:

Both Vouchers and CBHI are Highly Cost-effective

At a cost of $302 (Alfonso et al) per DALY averted for vouchers and $221 (most favorable) and $298 (most likely) per DALY averted for subsidy of CBHI, both interventions are highly cost-effective and virtually identical in their cost-effectiveness ratios. According to the World Health Organization, if the cost-effectiveness ratio is less than a country's per capita GNP, the intervention is highly cost effective. In the case of Uganda, this is $510 per capita (www.worldbank.org). On policy grounds, the subsidy of CBHI is more consistent with a broader policy supported by Uganda and other partner states in the East African community: expand social health protection through enrolling the population in universal health insurance. Insurance should also include outreach to encourage poor women to deliver at health facilities, transportation to and from health centers for deliveries, and incentives to health workers for increased volume and quality. Whereas vouchers create a separate mechanism for pregnant women, the subsidy of insurance could be done with a broader context of universal health insurance, partially subsidized, for the entire population.

Whereas most CBHI programs cover only medical services and not transportation, the voucher and SHU schemes also provide transportation coverage for a woman to go to a health center for delivery, and obstetrical transfers, if needed from a health center to a referral site. These are both very important services. We recommend that they become part of a system of subsidized CBHI.

Advance Towards Universal Health Coverage

The CBHI system has the advantage of advancing progress towards universal health insurance, a policy goal of all five partner states in the East African Community. Thus, donor subsidy of those programs serves a broader policy goal.

Develop Hybrid, Sliding Scale Programs for Charges to Clients

The programs would seek to enroll all pregnant women, with the enrollment fee based on a sliding scale. The poorest women would pay only a token fee; the most affluent would pay close to the actuarial cost of their services, and the intermediate group a partial amount. This would mirror the system in Rwanda, where households are classified by "ubudehe" level and the premium for CBHI (mutuelle) varies accordingly.

Include All Sectors

Include government, NGO and private-for-profit facilities and embrace key services for both access and quality. The access services are both normal and complicated delivery (upon medical indication by a neutral source of referral), boda-boda (motorcycle) or taxi transport for the delivery, and emergency ambulance transfer in obstetric emergencies.

Extend Quality Reviews

Use quality reviews to identify quality facilities, but also to offer training to facilities to upgrade and maintain quality, and incentives to the staff (particularly in government facilities) for meeting these quality standards.

Limit the Administrative Cost of CBHI and Vouchers

The administrative cost of both CBHI and vouchers should be carefully managed. Management by local organizations, such as Save for Health Uganda (SHU), may be more cost-effective than that by international non-governmental organizations, which are likely to have greater overhead costs. SHU is a local NGO that has maternal health insurance schemes in four districts that have been turned into CBHI schemes for the entire population.

It also has other CBHI schemes covering all age groups in five other districts. A possibility of using commercial health insurance schemes like Medical Link Company with a product called MILO (Medical Insurance for Low income groups) could also be useful. Health coop models offer additional lessons that could be valuable especially as part of a national health insurance scheme. Other private companies should be willing to discuss maternity health insurance with a financing agency. The inherent advantage is that these companies have a countrywide network of providers and information technology that can be used at a low additional cost.

Maintain Sustainable Designs

For sustainability of the programs, continue to actively involve the beneficiary communities, local leadership, entire health sector leadership (Ministry of Health, donors and civil society) in management of RHV and CBHI. The funding agency could gradually build capacity for the communities to manage or actively participate in the RHVs, CBHI, health coops and national health insurance scheme as one key step towards universal coverage.

Gain More Information

CBHI and RHV should be expanded with an experimental design, if possible, to provide more information about the updates and impact. This expansion could be done by a 3-arm cluster randomized design in which sub-counties are randomized among usual care (usual facilities and payment), CBHI and RHV. Costs, utilization, and outcomes would be measured in each arm, which should be preceded by strong baseline studies.

ACKNOWLEDGMENTS

The contribution of Daryl Martyris of USAID Uganda and Uziab Saya Management Science for Health Washington to the consultancy report on this work is appreciated.

REFERENCES

[1] World Health Organisation. 2014. *Website: Cost-effectiveness thresholds.* (Last accessed on10th October 2017). http://www.who.int/choice/costs/CER_thresholds/en.

[2] National Center for Biotechnology Information (NCBI). 2006. *Priorities in Health, Chapter 4 Cost-Effective Strategies for the Excess Burden of Disease in Developing Countries.* Washington, DC: The World Bank. Bookshelf ID: NBK10258. http://www.ncbi.nlm.nih.gov/books/NBK10258 (Last accessed on 8th December 2017).

[3] Ministry of Health. 2010. *The Second National Health Policy: Promoting People's Health to Enhance Socio-economic Development*. Kampala; MOHU.

[4] Ministry of Health. 2013. *Health Sector Performance Report 2012/13.* Kampala, MOHU.

[5] Okwero, P. et al. 2010. *Fiscal space for health in Uganda.* Washington DC, World Bank.

[6] KfW Entwicklungsbank. *Reproductive Health Voucher Programs in Kenya and Uganda.* KFW Position Paper 2011. Accessed at www.kfw-entwicklungsbank.de/Download-Center/PDF-Dokumente-Positionpapiere/2011 *Gesundheit-Voucher*_E.pdf, on 24 November, 2017.

[7] Population Council. 2013. *Evaluation of the Healthy Baby Program.* New York.

[8] Kanya, L. et al. 2014. Safe motherhood voucher programme coverage of health facility deliveries among poor women in South-western Uganda. *Health Policy and Planning*; 29 (Suppl1):i4–i11.

[9] Mazzilli, C. 2011. *The cost-effectiveness of a voucher programme for facility-based delivery in six districts of Western Uganda: A critical analysis*. London: Marie Stopes International, Unpublished.

[10] Basaza R., Pariyo G., Criel B. *What are the emerging features of community health insurance schemes in East Africa*?. Dove Medical Press Ltd. 2009; Volume 2: pp. 47-53.

[11] World Health Organization and UNICEF. 2012. *Building a Future for Women and Children: The 20120 Report. Countdown to 2015: Maternal, Newborn and Child survival.* Geneva, WHO.

[12] Alfonso, Y.N. et al. 2015. Cost Effectiveness analysis of a voucher scheme combined with obstetrical quality improvements: quasi experimental results from Uganda. *Health Policy and Planning*; 30(1):88-99.

[13] The New Vision. 2013. *Uganda's maternal death reduces - WHO report.* Online: https://www.newvision.co.ug/new_vision/news/1321806/ugandas-maternal-death-reduces-report; (accessed on 20th November 2017).

[14] Hogan M.M.C., et al. 2010. Maternal mortality for 181 countries, 1980-2008: A systematic analysis of progress towards Millennium Development Goal 5. *Lancet* 375:1609–1623. doi:10.1016/S0140-6736(10)60518-1.

[15] Uganda Bureau of Statistics (UBOS) and ICF International Inc. (2012). *Uganda Demographic and health Survey 2011*. Kampala, Uganda: UBOS and Calverton, Maryland: ICF International Inc. http://dhsprogram.com.pubs/pdf/FR 264.pdf. Uganda - Uganda National Household Survey 2002/2003

[16] UNDP. 2013. *Website*. Accessed from: http://hdr.undp.org/en/2013-report.

[17] World Health Organization. 2012. *Trends in Maternal Mortality: 1990 to 2010*. Geneva; WHO.

[18] Jain, A.K. 2011. Measuring the effect of fertility decline on the maternal mortality ratio. *Stud Fam Plann* 42: 247–260.

[19] Bellows, B.W. et al. 2013. A taxonomy and results from a comprehensive review of 28 maternal health voucher programmes. *Journal of Health Population and Nutrition*; 31(4) (Sppl2):S106-S128.

[20] Barros A.J.D. et al. 2012. Equity in maternal, newborn, and child health interventions in Countdown to 2015: a retrospective review of survey data from 54 countries. *Lancet* 379: 1225–1233. doi: 10.1016/S0140-6736(12)60113-5.

[21] Uganda Bureau of Statistics. 2015. *Uganda Population and Housing Census Report*. Kampala, UBOS.

[22] Kiwanukaa et al., 2008. Access to and utilization of health services for the poor in Uganda: a systematic review of available evidence. *Trans R Soc Trop Med Hyg*; 102(11):1067-74. doi: 10.1016/j.trstmh. 2008.04.023.

[23] Ekirapa-Kiracho et al. 2011. Increasing access to institutional deliveries using demand and supply side incentives: early results from a quasi-experimental study. *BMC International Health and Human Rights;* 11(Suppl 1):S11. https://doi.org/10.1186/1472-698X-11-S1-S11.

[24] Kanya, L. 2014. Safe motherhood voucher programme coverage of health facility deliveries among poor women in South-western Uganda. *Health Policy Planning*, 29(Suppl 1): i4–i11.

[25] Ministry of Health. 2013. *Health Sector Performance Report 2012/13*. Kampala, MOHU.

[26] Organization of African Unity. 2001. *Abuja declaration on HIV/AIDS, tuberculosis, and other related infectious diseases (OAU/SPS/ ABUJA/3):* http://www.un.org/ga/aids/pdf/abuja_declaration.pdf.

[27] Kyomugisha, E.L., et al. 2009. Strategies for sustainability and equity of prepayment health schemes in Uganda. *African Health Sciences*, 9(2). Accessible from: http://www.ajol.info/index.php/ahs/article/ view/48656.

[28] Orem, J.N. and C.M. Zikusooka. 2010. Health financing reform in Uganda. How equitable is the proposed National Health Insurance scheme? *International journal for equity in health*; 9, 23-23. Accessible from: http://www.biomedcentral.com/content/pdf/1475-9276-9-23.pdf.

[29] Kimani, J.K. et al. 2014. Determinants of health insurance ownership among women in Kenya: evidence from the 2008-09 Kenya demographic and health survey. *Int J Equity Health* 13: 27. doi:10.1186/1475-9276-13-27.

[30] Odeyemi, I.A.O. 2014. Community-based health insurance programmes and the national health insurance scheme of Nigeria: challenges to uptake and integration. *International Journal for Equity in Health;* 13:20. https://doi.org/10.1186/1475-9276-13-20.

[31] Basaza, R.K., Criel, B., and Van der Stuyft, P. 2010. Community health insurance amidst abolition of user fees in Uganda: the view from policy makers and health service managers. *BMC Health Services Research* 10.1:33 http:www.biomedcentral.com/1472-6963/10/33.

[32] Options Consultancy Service. 2013. *Options briefing paper on the role of vouchers and universal health coverage.* London, UK. (Last accessed on 8th December 2017). http://www.options.co.uk/about-options/news/355-options-briefing-paper-on-the-role-of-vouchers-and-universal-health-coverage.

[33] Shepard, D.S. et al. 2012. A controlled study of funding for Human Immunodeficiency Virus/Acquired Immunodeficiency Syndrome as resource capacity building in the health system in Rwanda. *American Journal of Tropical Medicine and Hygiene;* 86(5):902-907. Accessible from: http://www.ajtmh.org/cgi/reprint/86/5/902.

[34] Zeng, W. et al. 2014. Efficiency of HIV/AIDS health centers and the effect of community-based health insurance and performance-based financing on HIV/AIDS service delivery in Rwanda. *American Journal of Tropical Medicine and Hygiene* 90(4):740–746. (doi:10.4269/ajtmh.12-0697e).

[35] Rwiyereka, A.K. 2013. *Making Money Work for Mothers: A Quantitative and Qualitative Assessment of the Impact of Novel Health Financing Policies on Maternal Health Services in Rwanda.* (PhD Dissertation). Waltham, MA: Heller School for Social Policy and Management, Brandeis University.

[36] Gavagan, T.F. 2010. Effect of financial incentives on improvement in medical quality indicators for primary care. *J Am Board Fam Med;* 23(5):622-31. doi: 10.3122/jabfm.2010.05.070187.

[37] Grainger, C. et al. 2014. Lessons from sexual and reproductive health voucher program design and function: a comprehensive review. *International Journal for Equity in Health*; 13:33. Accessible from: http://www.equityhealthj.com/content/13/1/33.

[38] Obare, F., et al. 2016. *Increased coverage of maternal health services among the poor in western Uganda in an output-based aid voucher scheme.* Policy research working paper; 7709.

[39] Levin, A., McEuen, M., Dymatraczenko, T. et al. 2000. *Costs of maternal health care services in three Anglophone African countries.* Bethesda, MD: Partnerships for Health Reform Project, Abt Associates, Inc.

[40] Save for Health Uganda. 2014. *Annual Report 2013.* Kampala, SHU.

[41] The World Bank. 2014). *World Development Indicators.* http://wdi.worldbank.org/table/1.1 (Last accessed on 15th December 2017).

[42] Dorsey, G. et al. 2007. *Combination therapy for uncomplicated falciparum malaria in Ugandan children.* JAMA. 297:2210-2219.

[43] Zurovac D. et al. 2008. Malaria case-management under artemether-lumefantrine treatment policy in Uganda. *Malaria Journal*; 7:181 doi:10. 1186/1475-2875-7-181.

[44] Kohler, J. et al. 2012. The "*Insurance Effect": A statistical analysis of the relationship between health insurance and family planning in seven countries.* Abt Associates, Bethesda. Accessed at www.docstoc.com/docs/139458350/2012_12_03_FINAL_Family_Planning_and_Insurance_Report on 8 Dec. 2014.

In: The Journey …
Editors: Robert Basaza et al.
ISBN: 978-1-53618-323-8

Chapter 3

COMMUNITY HEALTH INSURANCE IN UGANDA: THE LONELY JOURNEY OF COMMUNITY HEALTH INSURANCE TO UNIVERSAL HEALTH INSURANCE COVERAGE IN UGANDA WITH A CASE STUDY OF RWANDA

Prossy K. Namyalo[1,*], David Ogubi[2] and Robert Basaza[3]

[1]Ndejje University, Faculty of Social Sceince, Uganda
[2]International Health Sciences University, Uganda
[3]Gudie Incubation Centre, Kira Municipality, Uganda and Uganda Christian University, MPHL Program

[*] Corresponding Author's E-mail: pnkiddu@gmail.com.

ABSTRACT

The paper aims at presenting the genesis and development of Community Based Health Insurance (CHI) and contributing knowledge to the development of universal health insurance in Uganda, a key strategy under universal health coverage in sustainable development goals.

A cross sectional descriptive and retrospective study of CHI schemes in Uganda was done. Data was obtained through the records of the CHI umbrella organization; Uganda Community Based Health Financing Association. Data extraction sheets were developed and used to analyze individual scheme records. This was complemented by literature review on CHI in Uganda, the region and beyond.

A majority of the schemes are found in Southern and Western Uganda with a few in the Central region. The Eastern and the Northern Districts are starting to form them. Currently, there is no regulatory instrument for CHIS but they are registered as either community-based organizations at district level or non-government organizations by the Registrar of Companies at national level. The community managed CHIs have majority of the beneficiaries. A comparative case study about Rwanda with a rather successful case and larger coverage (over 75% of Rwandas' 10 million people) is presented.

CHI schemes were started with donor support and do not have a legal framework for the last 22 years. They face several challenges such as poverty of the population, limited government buy-in and inadequate technical capacity by the promoters. This has affected expansion of the schemes both in enrolment and depth of the package. The schemes face a policy dilemma of promotion of contributory payment for healthcare amidst a policy of free healthcare by government. The future of CHI will depend on the design of the proposed National Health Insurance and the will of the political actors in Uganda to establish a prepayment system in line with other East African Community Partner States.

ABBREVIATIONS

CHI	Community Health Insurance;
NHIS	National Health Insurance Scheme;
IPD	In-Patient Department;
IRA	Insurance Regulatory Authority;
KDCHIS	Kabale Diocese Community Health Insurance Schemes;

MOH	Ministry of Health;
OPD	Out Patient Department;
PNFP	Private Not for Profit;
UCBHFA	Uganda Community Based Financing Association;
UHIC	Universal Health Insurance Coverage

INTRODUCTION

This chapter aims at presenting the genesis and development of Community Based Health Insurance (CBHI) and contributing knowledge to the development of universal health insurance in Uganda, a key strategy under universal health coverage in Sustainable Development Goals. It analyzes the historical precedent of CHIS in Uganda from inception to the present.

Community Based Health Insurance (CBHI) Schemes or simply CHI are a form of voluntary prepayment that are heterogeneous, built on solidarity features and are characterized by voluntary enrollment, have a fixed premium with a limited range of healthcare services and targets the informal sector [1]. CHI refer to non-profit health financing schemes and sometimes the term is used to discuss those initiatives that are formed with a primary aim of collecting healthcare risks. Different scholars and people refer to CHIS differently. In West and Central Africa for example, they are commonly called Mutual Health Organizations (MHO) or *mutuelles de sante' in French*. They are also referred to as micro-insurance scheme, medical aid societies or medical aid schemes [2, 3, 4]. Nevertheless, applying the basic principle of risk sharing and running on a non-profit basis are the common characteristics of all.

Starting at Kisiizi hospital in Rukungiri district in 1995 in a pilot form, CHIS in Uganda have expanded to 24 with a combined more than 152, 260 individual beneficiaries. Kisiizi hospital being the first CHIS, was started with support from Department for International Development of UK and government of Uganda funding. Later, other development partners including Bread for the World (BftW), Catholic Organization for Relief Development

Aid (CORDAID), and USAID, became key funders of organizations that promote and support CHIS. The start of CBHIS in Uganda was an attempt to explore other health financing mechanisms especially after the failure to pay user fees and hospitals failing to raise a running budget [1, 5, 6].

METHODOLOGY

This was a cross sectional descriptive and retrospective study of CHI schemes in Uganda. Data was obtained from records of an umbrella CHI scheme organization; the Uganda Community Based Health Financing Association. Data extraction sheets were developed and used to analyze individual scheme records. This was complemented by literature review on CHI in Uganda, the region and beyond. The review was done by the three authors. Both grey and published literature were considered. The literature search was mainly from PubMed and Google scholar and used snow ball technique for wider inclusion.

RESULTS AND DISCUSSION

Uganda Community Based Health Financing Association

CHIS formed an umbrella association in 1998; the Uganda Community Based Health Financing Association (UCBHFA) with the objectives of: 1) to coordinate all community based health financing initiatives in Uganda, 2) to promote community based health financing in Uganda, 3) to advocate and lobby appropriate support and health insurance policies on behalf of members practicing community based health insurance schemes, 4) to conduct relevant research on community based health financing, and 5) to provide technical and managerial support to enhance the skills of individual scheme staff to improve the implementation of community based health financing [5, 7].

Table 1. Community Health Insurance Schemes and their Location

CHI Scheme Promoter	Scheme name	Type of scheme	N° of people covered	Name of Health Care facility	Level	Ownership	District
1. Save for Health Uganda (SHU)	Munno mu Bulwadde Union of Schemes Organization (MBUSO)	Member managed	27,015	Bishop Ceaser Asili Hospital	Hospital	PNFP/UCMB	Luwero
				Kiwoko Hospital	Hospital	PNFP/UPMB	Nakaseke
				Nakaseke Hospital	Hospital	GOVT	Nakaseke
				Franciscan HC	HC 1V	PNFP/UCMB	Nakasongola
				St. Luke Namaliga HC	HC 1V	PNFP/UCMB	Luwero
				Holly Cross HC	HC III	PNFP/UCMB	Luwero
				St. Matia Mulumba HC	HC III	PNFP/UCMB	Luwero
				St Kizito HC - Natyole	HC III	PNFP/UCMB	Luwero
				Our Lady of Lourdes HC	HC III	PNFP/UCMB	Nakasongola
	Munno mu Bulwadde Union of Schemes Organization	Member managed	3,578	Ishaka Adventist Hospital	Hospital	PNFP/UCMB	Bushenyi
				Kitagata Hospital	Hospital	Government	Sheema
				Mushanga HC	HC III	PNFP/UCMB	Sheema

Table 1. (Continued)

CHI Scheme Promoter	Scheme name	Type of scheme	N° of people covered	Name of Health Care facility	Level	Ownership	District
				Hope Medical Centre/AMG Bugongi	HC III	PNFP/UPMB	Sheema
				Bitooma HC	HC III	PFP	Bushenyi
	Mubende Munno Mu Bulwade Union of Schemes Coordination Mechanism (MUSCOM)	Member managed	2,395	St Francis Community HC	HC IV	PNFP/UCMB	Mityana
				ST. Gabriel Mirembe Maria HC	HC III	PNFP/UCMB	Kasanda
				Bangi Maternity Home	HC II	PFP	Kasanda
				Holy Family Naluggi HC	HC II	PNFP/UCMB	Mityana
				Kitokolo Health HC	HC II	PNFP/UPMB	Kasanda
	SHU managed CHI Schemes (SCS)	Third party managed	352	Bishop Ceaser Asili Hospital	Hospital	PNFP/UCMB	Luwero
				Kiwoko Hospital	Hospital	PNFP/UPMB	Nakaseke
				Franciscan HC	HC IV	PNFP/UCMB	Nakasongola
				Kitovu Hospital	Hospital	PNFP/UCMB	Masaka

CHI Scheme Promoter	Scheme name	Type of scheme	N° of people covered	Name of Health Care facility	Level	Ownership	District
2. ICOBI	ICO-CARE	Service provider managed	6,200	Crescent Medical Centre	HCIII	PFP	Jinja
				SOS Medical Centre	HC III	PFP	Wakiso
				Bushenyi Medical Centre	HC III	PFP	Bushenyi
				Kabwohe Clinical Research Centre	HCIV	PFP	Sheema
				St Kaloori Lwanga - Nyakibaare Hospital	Hospital	PNFP/UCMB	Rukungiri
				Nyakisenyi HC	HCIII	PNFP/UCMB	Rukungiri
3. Kabale Diocese	Kabale Diocese Community Health Insurance Scheme (KDCHIS)	Member managed	16,380	Buhara HC	HCIII	PNFP/UCMB	Kabale
				Rushoroza HC	HCIII	PNFP/UCMB	Kabale
				Nyamwegabire HC	HCIII	PNFP/UCMB	Kanungu
				Nyamirama HC	HCIII	PNFP/UCMB	Kanungu
				Makiro HC	HCIII	PNFP/UCMB	Kanungu
				St Kaloori Lwanga - Nyakibaare Hospital	Hospital	PNFP/UCMB	Rukungiri

Table 1. (Continued)

CHI Scheme Promoter	Scheme name	Type of scheme	N° of people covered	Name of Health Care facility	Level	Ownership	District
				Kibirizi HC	HCIII	PNFP/UCMB	Rukungiri
				Nyakisenyi HC	HCIII	PNFP/UCMB	Rukungiri
				Nyarushanje HC	HCIII	PNFP/UCMB	Rukungiri
				Ndama HC	HCIII	PNFP/UCMB	Rukungiri
				Rwengiri HC	HCIII	PNFP/UCMB	Rukungiri
				Kitanga HC	HCIII	PNFP/UCMB	Rukiga
				Mutolere Hospital	Hospital	PNFP/UCMB	Kisoro
				Kinanira HC	HCIII	PNFP/UCMB	Kisoro
				Kishanje HC	HCIII	PNFP/UCMB	Rubanda
				Muko HC	HCIII	PNFP/UCMB	Rubanda
4. Kisizi Hospital	Kisizi Hospital Community Health Insurance Scheme	Service provider managed	40,500	Kisizi Hospital	Hospital	PNFP/UPMB	Rukungiri
5. Bwindi Hospital	E-quality scheme	Service provider managed	28,006	Bwindi Hospital	Hospital	PNFP/UPMB	Kanungu
6. Health partners Uganda (HPU)	Uganda Health Cooperatives (UHC)	Service provider managed	3,000	Comboni Hospital	Hospital	PNFP/UCMB	Bushenyi
				Mitooma Central Clinic	HCIII	PFP	Mitooma

CHI Scheme Promoter	Scheme name	Type of scheme	N° of people covered	Name of Health Care facility	Level	Ownership	District
				Nyakatsiro HC	HC III	PNFP/UCMB	Mitooma
	Western Ankole Diocese Health Cooperatives (WADHC)	Service provider managed	18,234	Katungu Mission Hospital Project	HC III	PNFP/UPMB	Bushenyi
7. Ishaka Health Plan	Ishaka Health Plan (IHP)	Member managed	1,600	Ishaka Adventist Hospital	Hospital	PNFP/UPMB	Bushenyi
				Kampala International University Teaching Hospital	Hospital	PFP	Bushenyi
8. Happy Health Insurance Scheme	Happy Health Insurance Scheme	Service provider managed	5,000	Happy Health Insurance Scheme Clinic	Health Centre II	PNFP	Ntungamo
TOTAL			152,260	49 facilities			

Data extraction by authors' from UCBHFA, 2018 records.

UCBHFA is registered as a national non-governmental organization with its offices in Kampala. The secretariat is run by hired technical staff while the governance is by member representatives. The association's supreme arm, the general assembly seats once every year. Currently, the association has over 25 members including schemes and organizations that promote schemes [5, 6, 7].

The majority of these schemes are found in Southern and Western parts of Uganda with a few in Central and Eastern regions. The Northern Districts have also started forming CHIS (Uganda does not have regional or provincial administration). Table 1 highlights the different schemes, districts where they are found and their promoters[1]. CHIS depend on better built solidarity features which are inherent in South Western and Western parts of the country in addition to relatively higher incomes. The Poverty report of 2014 presented that only 4.7% and 8.7% respectively of the population of Central and Western regions in Uganda that were not able to meet their basic needs, while their counterparts had 24.1% and 43.7% for Eastern and Northern respectively [5, 8, 24].

The Policy Framework of CHIS

Vision 2040 which is the futuristic planning framework for Uganda provides for universal health insurance as one of the pillars of developing to middle and upper-income country. In the East African region, Uganda allocates the lowest amount of money to health, compared to her counterparts. Private spending on health is highest in Uganda compared to her counterparts in the region (41% in Uganda compared the lowest in Rwanda at 28%). More so, Uganda has no specific health protection policy nor does it have a social health protection research agenda. In the absence of a specific health insurance act, regulation of health insurance is hinged on

---

[1] Under Kabale Diocese Community Health Insurance Schemes (KDCHIS), there are 6 individual schemes that are members of UCBHFA. 2. Health Partners though a member of UCBHFA, is not a scheme but rather supports cooperatives (technically and financially); thus making a total membership of 25.

the Insurance Amendment Act of 2011 which led to the establishment of the Insurance Regulatory Authority (IRA) of Uganda. The Act provides for schemes' regulation and any other premium-receiving institutions including CHIS. Currently, there is no regulatory instrument for CHIS but are rather registered as either community-based organisations at district level or non-government organisations by the Register of Companies [8, 9].

The National Health Policy 2010 counts on promoting sustainable alternative health financing mechanisms. One of the specific objectives of the Health Sector Development Plan 2015/2016 -2019/2020 is to increase financial risk protection of households. This is because direct out of pocket payments are estimated to be at 42% of the total health expenditure. One of the identified interventions to achieving this objective is formulating the required legislation, such as the NHIS Bill. The Uganda Ministry of Health (MOH) already has a draft NHIS bill and though it initially recognized CHI as one of schemes within the bigger NHIS, the new version is silent about the same [7, 8, 9, 10, 11].

Community Based Health Insurance Schemes Management

CBHIS in Uganda are mainly community initiatives and thus have an independent management from the facilities and founding organizations [5, 6, 12]. They are mainly of two types:

- Community managed: This is where an organized community establishes a healthcare fund and contracts healthcare providers of their choice to provide them services. It is owned by the community and majority of the CHI beneficiaries in Uganda joined this form. This form has the following characteristics:
  - Managed by community members
  - Community members elect their leaders to run the scheme affairs
  - Leadership is based on voluntarism
  - Heavily depend on solidarity and social cohesion features

  - Community or group is the insurer and it bears all the risks.
- Provider managed: Initiated and managed by the health facility to improve access to some categories of people, depending on the healthcare providers' objectives. In this case, the healthcare provider's role is two folded: that is healthcare service provision as well as managing the healthcare fund. The scheme is normally taken as a department within the hospital or health centre. It has the following characteristics:
  - Management of the scheme is by the healthcare facility staff
  - Healthcare provider is the insurer and bears the risk
  - Communities play a supplementary role in the day to day management of the schemes.
  - The provider is involved in the mobilization and recruitment of scheme members and collecting premiums.
- Third party managed: Here, the community bears the full risk but management is by another entity. They are not well developed in Uganda but organizations like Save for Health Uganda have started managing them.

Principles on which CHIS Are Built

Irrespective of the way they are managed, CHIS are built on a number of principles [1, 2, 4, 6].

- Voluntary membership: There is free entry and exit of members. People willingly join after understanding the CHI concept; and basing on their need and the healthcare products being promoted.
- Solidarity or pooling: Solidarity features of willingness among community members to contribute for a common challenge and sharing healthcare risks among themselves through pooling of resources are strong in CHIS.
- Democratic governance: The community makes decisions concerning their scheme. This principle denotes that the community

participates in making their internal regulations (constitution) and electing their own leaders. This principle is very important if any CHIS is to succeed.

- Not-for-profit: CHIS are formed without any intention of making profits. Even when there are surplus at the end of the financial year, they are kept as reserves to meet future unexpected obligations.

CBHIS Operations

How CBHIS Are Started

As highlighted in [5, 6, 12], CHIS in Uganda are mainly started in two ways. However, in whatever case, each has its own leadership structure and internal regulations. Firstly, an organization or health facility goes out to promote and form CHIS. When they start functioning, the promoting organization pulls out and the schemes continue by themselves. For the provider based, the health facility continues working with the schemes and managing them. In this case the promoting organization plays the roles of:

- Developing the benefit package and calculating the scheme premiums
- Supporting the schemes to formalize their relationship with the healthcare service providers
- Conducting studies that inform the activities of the schemes like feasibility, satisfaction surveys, medical audits, impact assessments among others
- Developing scheme promotional tools and promoting schemes within their catchment area
- Developing CHIS management tools and training users on them
- Giving technical advice whenever needed.

In the second form, the people or group starts its own CHI and in most cases, it's an additional service to what they are already doing. That is, a group is already in existence and involved in some development activities, but they add CHI to their activities. In this instance, they seek for technical guidance from CHIS promoting organizations like UCBHFA.

Enrollment

Irrespective of their category, all CBHIS target and enroll families or households and or groups. The household head is encouraged to pay for all his or her people in a family. However, given the extended nature of families in Uganda coupled with the fertility rate of women which is 6.2 [13], some schemes implement a range of 1-4 people. This means that the family joins with at least 4 members in case they cannot afford to pay for everyone at home. This is one method that may favor adverse selection in CHIS. For groups or schools, they are taken up if 60% of its members buy into and pay the CHIS premium [3, 4, 14, 15]. The details of enrollment into CHIS in Uganda from 2009 to 2018 are presented in Table 2.

Table 2. Trends of CHI enrollment in Uganda

Year	No of schemes	Total enrollment (individuals)
2018	25	152,260
2017	25	150,000
2016	24	150,000
2015	24	150,000
2014	24	152,743
2013	26	141,634
2012	24	165,216
2011	20	142,923
2010	18	133,722
2009	16	84,873

Authors pooled data from UCBHFA (2018).

Enrollment periods are specific to individual schemes and range from quarter, semester to annual. In the annual period for instance, members pay an annual premium and are therefore covered for a year after which they have to renew their membership or else their scheme coverage is stopped. It is the same way it works for the semester and quarter enrollment systems [5, 14, 15].

Depending on their terms of enrollment, schemes have a waiting period which varies from two weeks to three months. The waiting period is applied so as to minimize adverse selection; in this case, enrollment is of mainly sickly people. This period allows the scheme to prepare an identity card for the new member. The waiting period is the time between payment of the premium and receiving a membership card and thus entitlement to health care benefits. Fully paid up individuals and or families are issued with identity cards. These cards are either per person in a family or the whole family gets one card having pictures of all its family members. Some schemes just have a computerized system of identifying beneficiaries at the time of receiving the service [8, 14, 15].

None of the schemes charge the actuarially determined premium and this is due to affordability difficulties faced by the target population. Generally, a technically calculated premium would probably cost more than UGX 100,000/= per person per year with a good level of pooling. Since many cannot afford the actual premiums, CHIS end up charging adjusted premiums to fit onto 'target population's pocket'. Currently, CHIS charge between 12,000/= to 20,000/= (USD 3.00-6.00) per person per annum. The reduction in the charged premiums brings about a compromise on the benefit packages being promoted by the CHIS [5, 8, 15]. The schemes may provide reduced benefits or impose extra pay and thus:

- Charge a co-payment per episode at the point of service provision. The intention is to reduce patients frequenting the facilities which in the end might affect the CHI healthcare fund. This co-payment varies for outpatient department (OPD) and inpatient department (IPD). The latter being higher than the former. The co-payment amount might even go up to 40% of the paid annual premium [6, 8, 14, 15].

- Lower the benefit package to cover basic care which definitely reduces the bills and thus the consumption of the healthcare fund. The benefit package is sometimes lowered to only cover emergencies, IPD only, with a lot of exclusion in terms of chronic ailments, normal deliveries, and eye glasses, referrals to other facilities, among others [6, 8, 14, 15].
- Lower the ceiling per aliment. Most schemes cover their beneficiaries up to an average ceiling starting at UGX 100,000/= for IPD and UGX 50,000/= for OPD per episode. The ceiling amount is normally inclusive of the paid co-payment. Sometimes the ceiling is put on the number of times a family has to access care using the scheme fund. This is so on especially chronic ailments [5, 6, 15].

CHI Healthcare Reimbursement Arrangements

Health centres and the general wings of public hospitals were declared free at the point of getting services by the President with effect from March 2001. However, a dual system was maintained especially at hospitals. The private wing is for those who can afford to pay and a general wing for those who have no money. The CHIS that are provider based are promoted within either Private not for Profit (PNFP) or Private Facilities. For those that are community owned, they normally contract PNFP, Private or even public facilities (the private wing) for healthcare service provision [1, 8, 16].

CHIS especially the community managed use a number of reimbursement arrangements and this depends on the negotiations done at the time of contracting. The chosen method has an effect on administration, cost control and the quality of healthcare services. More than one reimbursement method can be present in a single relationship. Whatever the type of the scheme, the healthcare provider (treats) scheme members and later (normally at the end of the month), presents a bill to the scheme for payment. After confirming that the bill is correct, those in-charge of managing scheme's money then pay the bill. For provider managed, the bill is issued to the scheme manager who makes payments to the facility [5, 6,

17, 18]. Table 3 gives an explanation of the different forms of healthcare reimbursement arrangements that CHIS use.

Table 3. Different Reimbursement Arrangement Methods Used in CHIS

Method	Description
Fee for Service	This is where healthcare providers get paid for each type of treatment item they have provided scheme beneficiaries. That is a fee is charged for specific services. For example, consultation, laboratory and drugs.
Straight discount on charges	This is where a hospital submits a full claim but the CHI discounts it (according to the earlier agreed upon discount) before it pays.
Package pricing/Bundled charges/Flat fees	Even though in some literature this form is used for only OPD, some CHIS use it for both OPD and IPD. This is where the charges are bundled into a single charge and it reduces the challenges that come with unbundling. For example, consultations fees, laboratory fees and drugs costs charged as one single charge for OPD. Alternatively, a number of procedures might have been performed on a patient put the CHIS pay just a bundled fee. CHIS use healthcare providers' data to bundle the charges.

Source: Normand & Weber 1994, Kongstvedt, 2001 and UCBHFA, 2017.

Challenges Faced by CBHIS

Uganda's CHIS cover around 5%-10% of the people in their locations. Despite promotion of schemes since mid-1990s, membership in CHIS has remained low [5]. This slow growth has been attributed to the numerous challenges that CHIS face [1, 5, 7, 8, 14, 15]:

- Absence of policy and legal framework for CHIS which undermines the role of stakeholders in mobilizing communities and resources, despite the fact that some health policy makers see it as an option for financing healthcare thus a relevant health policy. Besides, CHIS have no accreditation body. In the absence of a professional accreditation body, scheme beneficiaries are not protected from any malpractice that may arise from the scheme and or their promoters.

Government's low support to the CHIS leads to poor utilization of social capital and local innovations.

- Long distances to the contracted service providers yet the nearer ones are public facilities. Close to three quarters (72%) of Ugandans are within a radius of 5km to a public or not for profit facility.
- Poor quality of care provided has raised concerns for a decade now. For example, they are understaffed, experience stock outs of medicines, inadequate funding and poor infrastructure and staff absenteeism. That is why Uganda has continued to register high catastrophic health expenses of 40% in 2017 from 5% in 2001, despite the free care in public facilities. People end up seeking care in private health units which charge user fees.
- Limited information about health insurance among the population which requires huge investment in health insurance education, recruitment and retaining beneficiaries. Most schemes cannot afford the cost of this investment. Yet there is evidence of poor understanding of the insurance principles by both the targeted communities and scheme managers.
- CHIS have limited financial resource base and this not only weakens their sustainability but also undermines the quality of healthcare services that the beneficiaries access which further limits coverage.
- CHIS require payment of a premium but the indigents cannot pay. Since there are no subsidies, even many of those that have some incomes cannot afford the annual premium. Eight out of ten people that have not joined the CHIS sight lack of money to pay as contribution/premium. This situation heavily impacts the CHIS in a number of ways; a number of them do compromise the basic benefit package by having a lot of exclusion, get low retention rates and in some cases, a full scheme fails to renew for another period.

CHIS CONTRIBUTION IN THE PROPOSED NHI SCHEME

CHIS Recognition in the Draft Bill

Uganda has no specific health insurance act; it's only through the Insurance Regulatory Authority (IRA) that provides for the regulation of any premium receiving institution. Currently, the regulation of CHIS has been excluded. IRA has left the matter of regulation of schemes to the health sector and there are no existing mechanisms. The health sector does not have an existing regulatory framework. It is anticipated that National Health Insurance scheme (NHIS) when put in place shall develop such regulatory mechanisms. Nonetheless, Uganda being one of the East African Country partner states committed to improve the social health protection for its people, it is making its first steps in developing a national health insurance scheme. Uganda through the Ministry of Health has since 2006 been drafting a National Health Insurance Scheme (NHIS). This bill was passed by the Cabinet and presented to Parliament. The NHIS bill currently excludes CHIS. The Ministry of Health is presently working out modalities of how a relationship can be marshalled out [8, 10].

The Role CHIS Would Play in the Proposed NHIS

Within the East African region, Uganda has the lowest population living below the poverty line compared to her counterparts in the region. This points to the fact that it has significant potential to increase enrollment in well-organized CHIS [8]. This implies that there could be a possibility that CHIS can be developed and expanded to the whole country like the case of Rwanda. For close to 22 years now since CHIS have been in existence, the promoters of these initiatives have a rich knowledge base on health insurance which persons developing the NHIS bill can tap into. This will benefit them since many Ugandans are said to have limited information on CHI. The critical mass of human resources in CHI initiatives will provide facts and lessons learnt upon which CHI guidelines can be developed. For example, CHIS have over a time evolved into unique operational models (the community and provider managed and now third party) and these provide valuable information for benchmarking and development of country-wide CHIS. Talking about universal insurance coverage, population coverage is very vital. A majority of Ugandans (80%) are in the informal sector (mainly unorganized), they are hard to organize and this therefore possesses difficulties in collecting premiums. Nonetheless, MOH can work with the existing CHI by empowering them both financially and policy wise to ensure that all Ugandans especially those in the informal sector are sensitized and enrolled into some form of health insurance hence achieving universal health insurance. The CHIS have over a time developed a local accreditation of facilities and service contract management systems upon which NHIS can draw inference and design an acceptable CHI model that is responsive to the 80% of the Ugandans [5, 13, 15].

Case Study 3.1: Nakaseke CHI Schemes in Uganda

This case study examined the prospects and challenges in 19 community health insurance schemes in Nakaseke District, Uganda. The level of education, occupation and household size were major determinants of membership into the schemes. In this case study, over half (69%) of the population enrolled in CHI schemes because they did not want to worry about money when they are sick. Distance to the registration centres and facilities and, operational barriers like delays in registration played significant effect against joining the schemes. Another outstanding reason for not joining was unaffordability of the premiums. The participants were generally satisfied with the performance of the scheme with notable fears especially on access to benefits. The schemes had a positive effect on the health seeking behaviour of the members. The scheme has improved the health seeking behaviour of the rural households with improved access to formal health services fortified with trained health workers. All of the insured mothers sought antenatal and postnatal care (89%) compared to 78% not insured. The non-insured delayed the visits to the health centres because of the high OOP problem endemic among them. Lack of insurance indeed could be contributing to deferment in seeking healthcare and noncompliance with treatment regime. Knowledge of how the scheme operates and the health insurance concept is still inadequate.

Adopted from – International Health Sciences University, MPH Thesis of Mr. David Ogubi (2015); "Assessment of Prospects and Challenges of Community Health Insurance in Nakaseke District, Uganda."

Case Study 3.2: The Contribution of CHI to UHIC in Rwanda

This case is developed from the East African Community social health protection report, annual report of MOH Rwanda on CBHI and other related studies (8, 19-22). It underscores the role of CBHIs in Rwanda's UHIC success. Starting formally in 1999, CBHIS existed informally and were functional in Rwanda from 1960 to the period before the genocide. After piloting three schemes in the three districts of Kyumba, Kabgayi and Kabutare and later conducting prospective studies, it was found out that CBHIS improved access and utilization of healthcare services of the people in the informal sector. From these results, the MOH developed the first '*mutuelle*' policy which aimed at strengthening them, organizing management structures and improving partnerships with all involved in the scheme. Besides this, the government went ahead to strategize and organized the establishment of CBHIS and more than 75% of the Rwandans' enrolled in CBHI scheme.

The CBHI law was expounded in 2010 (20 & 21) with a major aim of providing universal and equitable access to quality healthcare services for the Rwandan populace. CBHIS are administered at district level while coordination is at MOH level which is in the process of being transferred to Rwanda Social Security Board under Ministry for Finance. The day today running of the CBHIS is guided by the manuals on which all officials were trained. Managing CBHIS at district level does not only ease promotion of the concept especially in rural areas but also strengthens management capacities of the CBHIS systems.

Subsidizing the poor's premiums is one way the CBHIS have attracted more members to enroll, making a great contribution to Rwanda in achieving full (97%) universal health insurance coverage (8). People's direct contribution amounts to only 55% and co-payments total to 5%. Government makes a direct contribution that amounts to 21%, with development partners making 11% and other sources bringing in 8% (19). To ensure equity and solidarity among the members, a contribution system based on households' capacity to pay was introduced. Payments into the CBHIS are done in social economic stratification way basing on the household's wealth. This system being called "*Ubudehe*" program, categorizes people into three groups each paying a different amount of premium and a top-up in form of subsidy made. The indigents are therefore subsidized and their premiums paid for by government and development partners while others that have some income, pay according to what they can afford and still a top-up is made from government. With this mechanism, 24.8% of the population was able to enjoy health insurance which they would have otherwise never joined because they were identified as the poorest (20, 21 22, 23). Like the CBHIS in Uganda, Rwandan CBHIS renew their membership on an annual basis. To ensure that people renew and purchase more health insurance, sensitization is done every year. The annual sensitization which is normally done at the end of each CBHI financial year improves people's knowledge on the benefits and importance of purchasing health insurance.

Currently, the CHI schemes in Uganda face a policy dilemma of promotion of contributory payment for healthcare amidst a policy of free healthcare by government. More so, this is in an environment where the government intends to introduce a contributory NHIS. The current design of NHIS provides potential hope for enrolment of the informal sector and potential expansion of the CHIS. The prospects and challenges of select CHI schemes in Uganda are presented in a case study 3.1 and those of a neighbouring country Rwanda are in 3.2.

CONCLUSION

The CHI schemes in Uganda were started with donor support and do not have a legal framework for the last 22 years. They continue to face several challenges like poverty among the population, poor quality of services, limited government buy-in and inadequate technical capacity by the promoters.' This has affected expansion of the schemes both in enrolment and depth of the benefit package. Currently, the CHI schemes face a policy dilemma of promotion of contributory payment for healthcare amidst a policy of free healthcare by government. More so, this is in an environment where the government intends to introduce a contributory NHIS. The current design of NHIS provides potential hope for enrolment of the informal sector and potential expansion of the CHIS. The future of CHI schemes could depend on the design of the NHIS and the will of the political actors in Uganda to establish a universal prepayment system in line with other East African Community partner states. The Ugandan health sector will need an in-depth study to explore reasons why CHI schemes have not been developed and promoted in the Eastern and the Northern Districts of Uganda compared to the Central and South Western regions.

ACKNOWLEDGMENTS

The editors are grateful to Prof. Edgar Mulogo and Prof. Fred Bagenda of the Department of Community Health, Faculty of Medicine, Mbarara University of Science and Technology for proof reading and enriching this chapter.

REFERENCES

[1] Basaza K R, Criel B and Stuyft Van der V. 2010. Community health insurance amidst abolition of user fees in Uganda: the view from policy makers and health service managers. *BMC Health Services Research*, 10:33.

[2] Criel B, Atim C, Basaza R, et al. 2004. Community health insurance (CHI) in sub-Saharan Africa : researching the context. *Tropical Medicine and International Health*, volume 9 no 10 pp 1041–1043.

[3] Musau, Stephen N. 1999. *Community-Based Health Insurance: Experiences and Lessons Learned from East and Southern Africa. Technical Report No. 34*. Bethesda, MD. Partnerships for Health Reforms Project, Abt, Associates Inc.

[4] Carrin G. 2003. *Community based Health Insurance Schemes in Developing Countries: facts, problems and perspectives*, Discussion Paper. Geneva, WHO.

[5] Uganda Community-Based Health Financing Association: *Path to Better Health.* 2018. www.ucbhfa.org (last accessed on 10th January 2018).

[6] Derriennic Y, Wolf R and Kiwanuka-Mukiibi P. 2005. *An assessment of Community Based Health Financing Activities in Uganda.* Bethesda, MD: The Partners for Health Reform *plus* Project, Abt Associates Inc.

[7] Uganda Community Health Financing Association. 2014. *Strategic Plan 2013/2014 -2017/2018.* Kampala, Uganda.

[8] East African Community. 2014. *Situational Analysis and Feasibility Study of Options for Harmonization of Social Health Protection Systems. Towards Universal Health Coverage in the East African Community Partner States*. Arusha, Tanzania.

[9] Ministry of Health. 2015. *Health Sector Development Plan 2015/16 - 2019/20*. Kampala, Ministry of Health, Uganda.

[10] Ministry of Health. 2019. *The National Health Insurance Bill.* Kampala, Ministry of Health, Uganda.

[11] Ministry of Health. 2010. *The second Health Policy*. Kampala, Ministry of Health, Uganda.

[12] Centre for International Development and Research. 1999. *Report on the 'Community Based Health Insurance'* – Regional Conference in Kampala, Uganda.

[13] Uganda Bureau of Statistics. 2014. *Statistical Abstract*. Kampala, Uganda Bureau of Statistics, Uganda.

[14] Basaza K R, Criel B and Stuyft Van der V. 2007. Low enrolment in Ugandan Community Health Insurance Schemes: Underlying causes and policy implications. *BMC Health Services Research,* 7:105.

[15] Uganda Community Health Financing Association. 2014. *Report on Consultations with CHI scheme managers, Ishaka Municipality, Bushenyi district.* Kampala, UCBHFA.

[16] Save for Health Uganda 2014. *Annual Report*. Kampala, Uganda.

[17] Normand, C. And A. Weber. 1994. *Social Health Insurance: A guide for planning*. Geneva: World Health Organization.

[18] Kongstvedt R. Peter. 2001. *The Managed Health Care Handbook – Fourth Edition*. Maryland: An Aspen Publication.

[19] Ministry of Health. 2012. *Annual Report: Community Based Health Insurance.* Government of Rwanda.

[20] Lu C. et al. 2012. Towards Universal Health Coverage: An Evaluation of Rwanda Mutuelles in Its First Eight Years. *PLoS ONE* 7(6): e39282. doi: 10.1371/journal.pone.0039282.

[21] Makaka A, Breen S & Binagwaho A. 2012. Universal health coverage in Rwanda: a report of innovations to increase enrolment in

community-based health insurance. *Lancet:* DOI: http://dx.doi.org/10.1016/S0140-6736(13)60293-7.

[22] Dhillon S. R. et al. 2012. The impact of reducing financial barriers on utilization of primary health care facility in Rwanda. *Global Public Health*: 7(11): 71-86.7.

[23] Shimales A. 2010. Community Based Health Insurance Schemes in Africa. African *Development Bank: Working Papers Series*, No. 120.

[24] Ministry of Finance, Planning and Economic Development. 2014. *Poverty Status Report 2014: Structural Change and Poverty Reduction in Uganda*. Economic Development Policy and Research Development, Kampala, Uganda.

In: The Journey …
Editors: Robert Basaza et al.
ISBN: 978-1-53618-323-8

Chapter 4

HEALTH COOPERATIVES IN UGANDA: WHAT ARE THE EXPERIENCES AND LESSONS FOR DEVELOPMENT OF UNIVERSAL HEALTH INSURANCE?

Britt Alexandra Cruz and Jennifer Wenborg*
Health Partners, US

ABSTRACT

Health cooperatives are an important solution to health care challenges in developing countries because they incentivize members to seek care early and providers to keep members healthy and improve quality of care. The purpose of this chapter is to provide strategies and lessons learnt from cooperative health financing in Uganda in order to enable health stakeholders to increase access to care while improving health outcomes. This chapter also aims at helping governments in similar context to design efficient and effective universal health care systems.

* Corresponding Author's E-mail: Britt.A.Cruz@healthpartners.com.

Methods

The sources of literature have been performance reports from HealthPartners Uganda and USA and published literature from similar schemes. The authors and institutional experience have been used to identify and pull literature and other relevant information on this topic.

Discussion and Lessons for the Health Sector

Studies show that in addition to seeking care sooner, health cooperative members in Uganda adopted more preventive healthy behaviors like washing hands and sleeping under long lasting insecticide treated mosquito nets compared to non-members. Providers who offer cooperative services enjoyed increased cost recovery due to reduced bad debt. The member-owned structure empowered beneficiaries to take control of their health and to demand quality services from their care providers.

Conclusion

By applying these lessons, governments can avoid common pitfalls and scale up systems to benefit all stakeholders with a focus on the informal sector as part of broader national health insurance scheme.

Abbreviations

BOD	Board of Directors;
CBHI	Community Based Health Insurance;
CFI	Certificate of Financial Implications;
EAC	East African Community;
LMIC	Low and Middle-income Countries;
MOU	Memorandum of Understanding;
NGO	Non-Governmental Organization;
NHIS	National Health Insurance Scheme;
OOP	Out-Of-Pocket Payment;
RCMS	Rural Cooperative Medical Scheme;

UMASIDA	Umojawa Matibabukwa SecktaIsiyo Rasmi Dar es Salaam (Dar es Salaam Association for Health Care Services in the Informal Sector);
UGX	Uganda Shillings;
USD	United States Dollars.

INTRODUCTION

This chapter depicts the establishment of health cooperatives in Uganda and documents the experiences and lessons for development of universal health care in Uganda and other low and middle-income countries on the journey to universal health insurance coverage. The chapter begins with the history of health cooperatives in Uganda followed by lessons learnt in structure, management and finance. Strengths and vulnerabilities of cooperatives are introduced followed by factors that determine success. The chapter then delves into the design and lessons learnt from similar health insurance models in China, Rwanda, Tanzania and Ghana. It concludes with recommendations for stakeholders and governments to design and launch self-sustaining health insurance schemes and universal health care systems.

Founded as a health cooperative in 1957, HealthPartners is the largest consumer governed health insurance organization in the United States. In 1997, HealthPartners President was approached by Land O'Lakes, an international dairy cooperative development organization, regarding challenges they were seeing in Uganda. Dairy cooperative members were falling sick and selling their only income generating asset, a dairy cow, to seek treatment. HealthPartners worked with local stakeholders to adapt the member-owned cooperative model to meet provider and member needs in rural Uganda. Scott Aebischer, Senior Vice President, has been leading the health cooperative development effort in Uganda ever since. About 50 health care providers and over 43,000 members in Uganda are benefitting from health cooperative membership and the numbers are growing every month [1]. From the beginning, HealthPartners goals were ambitious; the model had to be self-sustainable; member premiums had to be low enough for the informal sector to afford yet high enough for providers to recover treatment costs plus a small surplus to continuously improve quality.

Health care systems in the United States and throughout the world often unintentionally incentivize overtreatment. The National Health Insurance Fund in Ghana is struggling to pay claims within 90 days because the repercussion for over-reporting is difficult to effect in real time. In China, 2,000 years ago, health workers were only paid when their patients were healthy. When people fell sick, the health worker had to treat them so they would be healthy again and could resume payment. HealthPartners was committed to making sure the health cooperative model incentivized providers to keep members healthy while incentivizing members to seek care sooner [2].

Local customs can exacerbate health challenges. In Uganda, women do not often have access to money to pay for health care yet they make most of the health care decisions for themselves, their children and for men. Delays to seek care are dangerous especially for pregnant women and children under five where malaria is endemic and clean water is hard to find. In health cooperatives, members pay a small premium periodically and can seek care when they need it without fear of high bills. Early treatment seeking reduces the length and severity of illness, consequently reducing time lost from work or school. When patients seek care early, they are less expensive to treat and recover faster. The health cooperative model is an important initiative to improve health outcomes because providers make more money when members are healthy. Studies show that in addition to seeking care sooner, health cooperative members in Uganda adopted more preventive healthy behaviors like hand washing and sleeping under long lasting insecticide treated mosquito nets, compared to non-members. Providers who offer services to cooperative members enjoyed increased cost recovery due to reduced bad debt [3, 4].

The member-owned structure empowers members to take control of their health and to demand quality from their care providers. The challenge is for providers and members to learn and remember how to sustain the benefits of their partnership. Both parties must fulfill roles and responsibilities, like members paying premiums on time and care providers checking identity cards (ID) before charging treatment costs to the cooperative. Where the partnership is well managed, studies show providers enjoy significantly higher cost recovery and invest in their facility to improve the quality of care. Where roles are not filled, free rider challenges arise. Free riders are people who do not pay premiums but attempt to charge care to the cooperative. If a provider does not make identity cards before a group joins, they cannot identify who has paid and who has not. Any time there is a loophole like this, word spreads fast and provider cost recovery goes down as friends pose as "members" or members "drop out" and seek to pay only the small premium when they fall sick. When there is no shared risk, insurance will not be sustainable. By applying these lessons, governments can avoid common pitfalls in national health insurance scheme design.

Health cooperatives are an ideal model to increase access to care for the informal sector as part of a broader scheme where formal sector premiums offset the cost of care for the impoverished. Health cooperatives engage the informal sector in partnership directly with their care provider. This increases member awareness of their rights and empowers them to advocate for quality care without increasing the government's burden of management costs, expenses and time-consuming claims processes [3, 4, 5].

By any means of delivery, health insurance aims at attaining three outcomes: 1) curb cost escalation, 2) improve the quality of care and 3) increase coverage. In all cases, it does so by sharing risk. Many people invest resources, but few fall ill, so the pooled resources cover costs of treating the ill [1]. That said, the means of delivery—or health insurance model—can vary significantly and the model used defines the overall experience, affordability and quality of care of the end-user. Each model has its own distinct objectives, challenges and benefits [1, 5].

There are three basic means of delivery into which health insurance can be divided [3]. The first is government-sponsored health insurance or public insurance, which aims to provide health insurance as part of a larger welfare goal. Generally, premiums are set in accordance with income, rather than health risk. Government health insurance is often considered a social good and can be either mandatory or volunteer-based. While government insurance may be affordable, it is most often provided only to the formal sector, given the logistical and financial challenges associated with collecting premiums from the informal sector.

The second category is private (for-profit) health insurance. While private players want to provide good quality services, their ultimate goal is to earn a profit. Membership is voluntary and premiums are based on health risk. Higher risk requires higher premiums. Those who can pay for the best services can access them. Profits return to the private entity. Private health insurance plays a minimal role in sub-Saharan Africa and will likely continue to play a minimal role for the foreseeable future, due to lack of economic resources [4, 5, 6].

Community-based health insurance (CBHI) serves those in the informal sector with fewer resources who are not served by government or private insurance [3, 4, 5]. CBHI can take many forms ranging from one local provider working with a small group of community members, as is the case in many sub-Saharan African countries, to nationwide, well-integrated systems found in China or Rwanda [3, 4, 5, 6]. Health cooperatives are one form of CBHI. Cooperatives are independent businesses, owned and run by and for their members. They are formed most often in response to a problem in the market--in this case, lack of insurance option for the informal sector. By pooling resources, cooperative members have more bargaining power to affect the prices and quality of their health care [1, 5, 7].

Cooperatives ascribe to seven universal principles:

1. Open and voluntary membership
2. Democratic control
3. Member's economic participation
4. Autonomy and independence
5. Education, training and information
6. Cooperation among cooperatives
7. Concern for community

These values form the basis for a health cooperative that is committed to self-help, self-responsibility, democracy, equity and solidarity. These principles guide the decisions of cooperative leadership and form a cooperative that is unique in its concerns for the community, educating its membership, sharing knowledge, and ensuring its members' needs are met by directly connecting providers with members. Since health cooperatives are a subcategory of CBHI which is distinctive mostly in its administration, literature specific to health cooperatives is often absorbed into the larger conversation about CBHI [1, 4, 6].

THE METHODOLOGY

The chapter literature is drawn from both grey and published sources. These are performance reports and records from HealthPartners Uganda and USA, and published literature from similar schemes. The authors and institutional experience have been used to identify and pull literature and other relevant information on this topic.

FINDINGS AND DISCUSSION

This section addresses the strengths, vulnerabilities and factors that determine the success of health cooperatives.

Strengths of the Health Cooperative Model

The following characteristics give CBHI models certain benefits over their counterparts in the government/public or private for-profit insurance markets [3, 4, 5, 6, 7]:

1. Premiums are moderate: Because premiums are set to cover the costs of treating patients, rather than to maximize profits, they are often lower than premiums set by private insurers.

2. Covers the informal sector: Premiums are collected via community-based mechanisms. Formal collection mechanisms are not necessary and as such coverage can easily be expanded.
3. Reduces risk of financial catastrophe: While this benefit is found in all health care models, the risk of financial catastrophe is often heightened in the informal sector, where incomes tend to be lower and less consistent; and high health care costs pose a greater danger of impoverishment.
4. "Bottom-up" development: Often used in locations where government investment in health care is low, health cooperatives can protect the vulnerable without direct investment from governments. Schemes are formed organically by those who will manage them, building ownership and accelerating scheme development, rather than waiting for government mandates or regulations.

There are additional benefits that are particular to health cooperatives, many of them social in nature:

1. Empower disenfranchised populations: Because health cooperatives are managed at the local-level, communities are empowered to make choices about where they will access care, how much it should be valued, and they can drive the quality of care. Member owners are also educated and trained as a matter of cooperative principle and good management, building member and provider social capital as a result of their affiliation with the cooperative.
2. Empower women: Women are the primary health care decision-makers in their households. Prepaid cooperatives allow women to access services for themselves and their families without having to ask permission or wait to collect money for out-of-pocket fees from their partners. Additionally, cooperative law requires female participation in governance, giving women a voice in shaping and managing the model that they may not otherwise have.

3. Profit remains in local clinics and communities: Provider surpluses from the cooperative can be used to directly invest in clinics and indirectly in cooperative management. Providers are able to reinvest profit to improve quality of care for everyone. Members understand that by participating in the cooperative, they are supporting their community and building the quality of their own health care.
4. Prepayment reduces administrative costs: The cooperative model is not claims-based, which would require extensive administrative systems and personnel to operate. The claims process can unintentionally incentivize over-reporting whereas prepayment incentivizes providers to keep members healthy so they incur lower treatment costs. The system of prepayment buys packages of care, not individual units, creating an administratively streamlined process that reduces administrative costs.
5. Improved health: Since members prepay for services, providers are incentivized to keep members healthy. Members are more likely to access services earlier if they fall sick and their incidence of illness is lower than patients who pay out-of-pocket.

Vulnerabilities of Health Cooperatives

Paradoxically, many of the same benefits that make health cooperatives attractive make the model particularly vulnerable. Because they are community-managed voluntary schemes into which stakeholders pay minimal premiums through informal payment mechanisms based largely on community solidarity, health cooperatives are exposed to challenges of financial sustainability, poor management, and lack of political support. These challenges have been widely documented in the literature. A few of the most cited are discussed [7, 8, 9, 10, 11].

- Financial sustainability: Premiums are often paid through community members who volunteer their time. Collection methods are most often informal. Whereas the formal sector can rely on taxes or salary deductions, the informal sector has no such organized means. They also have less capacity to create efficient documentation strategies, making records less accurate and often overlooked.
- Adverse selection: The model is voluntary, which means those who sign up are often the sickest. Without a means of reducing adverse selection (organizing premium payments by group, for example) and ensuring a large enough (and healthy enough) risk pool, the model can easily become financially unsustainable.
- High levels of poverty: Prioritizing health care requires an active decision to prioritize health along with other necessities.
- Weak managerial capacity: Because health cooperatives are often managed by community members in rural areas, management capacity in finance, human resources, monitoring and evaluation and other areas of critical importance to health insurance sustainability are often weak.
- Lack of legal and regulatory framework: Since health cooperatives may operate outside government systems, they are not always regulated like other insurance models. This means that schemes may not have legal protections like equal access to markets, voluntary membership, equal treatment of cooperatives and the right to due process. Lack of regulation can endanger the foundation of the scheme.
- Low enrolment rates: In general, health cooperative schemes are small, due to lack of resources and lack of knowledge or understanding of the model. Without the ability to cross-subsidize (wealthy with the poor, healthy with the sick) and link the poor to additional financing help, health cooperative enrolment will likely stay relatively low.

Factors that Determine Success of Health Cooperatives

Experts are beginning to coalesce around the idea that the root cause of the health cooperative weakness is its isolation from formal health financing mechanisms and from larger provider networks and benefit packages [10]. Linking health cooperatives to formal financing mechanisms and larger provider networks would address many of these identified vulnerabilities. Additional factors that determine the success of CBHI models are:

- Perceived quality of care;
- Ability of the model to respond to people's needs;
- Government commitment—regulations and a commitment to subsidize premiums for the poor; and
- Need for health cooperatives to form networks [11].

Wang and Pielemeier (2012) build on the idea of linking health cooperatives, expanding risk pools and ensuring government commitment in their framework for cooperative success. They essentially argue that only those models that achieve nationwide status--with strong government support, national coverage, formalized financing mechanisms--are sustainable in the long-term and will contribute to universal health care in low income countries. According to their approach, the key to success is integrating the characteristics of tax-based financing and social insurance schemes into cooperative development.

The following are characteristics of cooperatives at three evolutionary stages [1, 3, 5, 7, 12]:

1. Generic model
    - Pure grassroots, community-initiated, and managed models
    - Usually small and fragmented
    - Without legal and operational support and guidance from the government

2. Enhanced model
   - Recognized and supported by the government, but not well articulated as part of the broader government health finance policy/strategy
   - Government resources injected into these schemes to include the poor
   - Better networking among schemes (e.g., a federation)
   - Better capacity in negotiating and dealing with service providers
3. Nationwide model
   - Strong government commitment that brings stewardship, legislation, and funding support
   - Professional support and control of abuse and fraud
   - National coverage
   - Schemes are linked with other risk pooling and other national financing mechanisms.

There are a few examples of success of the type Wang and Pielemeier describe at the national level. Examples explained later are Rwanda and China. The authors note that while the generic cooperative model can be successful at reducing financial vulnerability in the short term; unless it evolves into an enhanced and eventually nationwide scheme, cooperative schemes will ultimately succumb to the weaknesses presented in this chapter.

What Is the Situation of Health Cooperatives in Uganda?

In Uganda, CBHI schemes including health cooperatives generally fall into the 'generic' category, to use Wang and Pielemeier's terminology. Schemes are relatively small and fragmented. They have no legal support from the government and they are managed at the community level. There have been efforts to network schemes—notably with the creation of the

Uganda Community Based Health Financing Association in 1998—and the government recognizes that the schemes exist. However, without government resources and legal support, the effort to evolve cooperatives and CBHI has not been widely successful. Nation-wide, an estimated 150,000 people are involved in some CBHI or cooperative scheme [9, 13]—coverage of only 5-10% of the eligible populations in the locations where they are found.

Uganda is ripe for wider cooperative development. Of all East African countries (EAC), Uganda has the lowest percentage of its population below the poverty line (27%), suggesting an ability to pay premiums for health cooperative coverage. The government contributes only 8.7% of its budget to health, the lowest in the region—despite having signed onto the Abuja Declaration over 15 years ago, which proposed a 15% baseline allocation. As a result of low government expenditure, household expenditure on health accounts for 40% of total health expenditures. High Out-of-Pocket (OOP) costs force many into poverty. In 2006, 2.3% of all households were newly impoverished as a result of OOP spending and the proportion of households that incurred catastrophic health expenditure was 28%. The wide gap between government spending and household spending, plus the potential for households to contribute to health care costs, suggests a much larger role for health cooperatives as a means of mitigating risks associated with high OOP costs [14, 15, 16].

Despite the low financial contributions to the health sector, the Ugandan government is pushing its agenda to provide universal health care through its proposed national health insurance scheme (NHIS). For the last fifteen years, the Ministry of Health (MOH) has been trying to initiate a health financing scheme that would diversify health care financing and provide financial risk protection. The National Health Insurance Bill 2019 was passed by the Cabinet and tabled in Parliament. The launch of the scheme will depend on when MOH obtains approval by the Parliament and successful launch by the government [17].

The bill recognizes CBHI as one of three sub-schemes in the NHIS—along with social health insurance and private commercial health insurance. While recognition of health cooperatives as a critical component of the

NHIS is a boon to CBHI schemes in the country, the legal and regulatory framework to allow them to flourish is still lacking, as is any explanation of how they will be organized, financed or adequately integrated into the NHIS [17]. Approximately one third of all CBHI scheme members in Uganda belong to a health cooperative where training was provided by HealthPartners. Membership in health cooperatives, as of July, 2017, was about 43,000. HealthPartners has been in Uganda for twenty years providing support in the form of technical advice to community groups and providers looking to form health cooperatives. In that time, it has gathered a substantial foundation of knowledge about how health cooperatives can be organized and financed sustainably [16]. These lessons are critical to understand as Uganda determines how to move forward with CBHI as a major component of the NHIS. The next section will explain the health cooperative scheme structure and financing and then identify lessons learned that are useful in conceptualizing a Ugandan NHIS.

Health Cooperative Scheme Structure, Management and Funding

Cooperatives are formed when groups—employee groups, funerary groups, schools—come together to prepay for health care services. Cooperatives are managed by democratically elected boards of directors (BODs), which have autonomy and independence to make decisions they believe are in the best interest of their members. The BODs manage the relationship between provider and members to ensure that the partnership delivers affordable, quality services to members while providing significantly higher cost recovery for providers. BODs are responsible for communicating and educating members, collecting and analyzing data, financial tracking, holding annual general meetings, expanding membership and advising providers that are failing to reach surplus. The BODs are typically volunteers and where financially feasible, they hire staff to carry out some of these roles. Cooperative group leaders collect premiums and lists of members who have paid their quarterly premiums to give to providers [1, 19, 12].

Health care providers are responsible for administration—enrolling new groups in the cooperative, providing them with identification, collecting lists of paid members, ensuring identification is always checked at the clinic, and tracking and analyzing cooperative performance data. They also play a key role in the success of health cooperatives and establish strong partnerships in the community through their cooperative efforts [1, 12, 19]. Most cooperative members pay approximately 5,000 UGX ($1.38 USD) per quarter to access basic services. Benefit packages vary between cooperatives, but in general, they cover preventive services, non-chronic care, maternity and laboratory services, and generic prescriptions. Members are required to pay membership dues at the beginning of each year and upon joining the cooperative, as a means of ensuring their economic participation, capitalizing the cooperative and dis-incentivizing drop outs. Members are also required to make copayments at the point of service to reduce moral hazard. The scheme is prepayment based, not claims based, so all premiums go to the provider to cover the costs of treatment. Providers then pay 10% of their surplus back into the cooperative's reserve fund at the end of the year to cover costs of running the cooperative. During the start-up phase, HealthPartners provides technical advice, training and minimal, results-based investments to offset transportation and facilitation costs. Emphasis is placed on training cooperative governance and members, since they are owners of the cooperative [1, 12, 19].

Funds for health cooperatives come from paid premiums, member dues and provider surpluses. HealthPartners does not provide reinsurance or subsidies, since doing so reduces the provider's incentive to properly manage its scheme [1].

Cooperatives are networked together through inter-cooperative meetings whereby cooperatives learn from each other, share promising practices and unsuccessful strategies in order to improve performance. Ongoing efforts continue to be made to create an apex organization for cooperatives and other CBHI schemes, but lack of capacity, financing and government support have proven substantial barriers. The impact of health care cooperatives on their members and providers was measured in 2015 by an external consultant. Members were generally healthier than non-members. They were more likely to take up preventive behaviors (washing hands, sleeping under mosquito nets), more likely to access early treatment and less likely to fall ill. Members were also better protected from high health care costs. They were less likely than patients paying out of pocket to borrow money, pay on credit or sell assets to pay for health care. Providers were also shown to benefit considerably from the partnership. Where patients were paying out of pocket, health care providers surveyed were likely to lose money (1,565 UGX/$0.50 USD). This was due to high numbers of patients who could not pay their bills. However, when treating cooperative members, providers were likely to make approximately 20,000 UGX ($6.38 USD), after accounting for treatment costs [1, 12, 14, 19, 21].

Lessons Learned

Health Cooperative Structure and Management

These lessons are drawn from international experience; work in sub-Saharan Africa and Uganda's local experience [1, 9, 10, 11, 12, 16, 19, 20]:

1. Cooperatives are businesses: Members and providers join together to create a mutually beneficial partnership. Both parties must see gains (either financial or health) in order to continue investing in the business. Once a cooperative is no longer meeting the needs of its members, it is no longer a sustainable business model.
2. Member control: Cooperatives require democratic governance as a principle. Members democratically elect a Board of Directors, whose primary role is to ensure a fair and mutually beneficial relationship between members and providers. BODs are responsible for setting premiums that are affordable for members while allowing providers to make surpluses so they can reinvest in their services. The ability of members to influence premiums and quality of care

empowers them to take control of their health care and identify ways for providers to improve services.

3. Shared risk between providers and members: Providers accept risk when they decide to accept prepayment for future care. Members accept risk when they decide to pay for treatment they may or may not need. Both parties win when premiums are affordable and total treatment costs are covered by premiums paid.
4. Group enrollment, not individual: In order to reduce the risk of adverse selection, cooperatives are encouraged to enroll groups, not individuals. Enrolling groups increases the pool of healthy individuals to offset the sick individuals. No health insurance model can survive without an adequate risk pool. In the model advocated by HealthPartners, individuals who choose to enroll must pay the equivalent of an entire family's premium to offset the additional potential cost of that individual.
5. Capable management: To sustainably operate a health cooperative, management must be able to collect and analyze data, ensure financial solvency, provide transparent governance, meet the needs of the members, and communicate with members to ensure continued buy-in. Most cooperatives are run by volunteer boards, who must receive adequate training. It is highly recommended that boards hire professional staff to support them in achieving all necessary objectives.
6. Identification: A major problem that will almost always lead to provider deficits is failure to delineate members from non-members. A cooperative must have an adequate system to identify those who have paid from those who have not. A policy of paying out of pocket must be enforced for all those who have not paid into the cooperative. Free-riders—those who are not paid members of the cooperative but access services under cooperative rates—will quickly reduce provider cost recovery.
7. Data collection and analysis: A cooperative works only if there is a balance between premiums paid and treatment costs incurred. In order to track the balance, providers and cooperatives need to collect

and analyze these data points on a regular basis. Cooperatives need to know who has paid, how much, and when they are due to pay again. They also need to know how much a provider is spending to treat cooperative patients to ensure premiums are covering treatment costs. Where there are deficits, the data can be consulted to determine if there is a problem with, for example, free-riders, an outbreak of disease, or if there is truly a problem with the cost balance.

8. Build upon existing health sector infrastructure: Building parallel structures (clinics, staff, and management) can be sustainable for a short period of time, but without continued investment, these structures eventually collapse. That is why it is so important to work within the defined infrastructure to strengthen existing systems, since they are likely to remain regardless of outside investment. Building on existing infrastructure also allows for leveraging local cultural norms and knowledge retention.
9. Intrinsic quality incentive: Members are often able to choose their provider in the cooperative model, which encourages providers to improve their quality to maintain a business partnership. As providers increase cost recovery and make a small profit, they are able to reinvest in their facilities so that they can improve their overall quality of care while retaining and expanding membership. As a general rule, when managed properly, rising membership leads to rising surpluses.
10. A network of cooperatives is stronger than individual cooperatives: Cooperatives face similar challenges and can gain significant knowledge and learn about promising strategies by talking with each other. While it is often difficult to justify the cost of getting together in person, there are many technologies that allow rapid knowledge sharing. HealthPartners has found WhatsApp to be a particularly useful tool for cooperative staff to share updates and answer each other's questions.
11. An umbrella or apex organization is required for long-term sustainability: HealthPartners and other donor funded organizations

can assist in providing technical assistance, training and capital initially. But cooperatives have fluctuating needs, changes in leadership and management and expansion opportunities over the course of their lifetimes, for which they may need continued technical support. A locally-run apex organization would have the capacity to provide the technical advice and training necessary to ensure continued success of cooperatives.

12. Communication: Cooperative members own their cooperative. In order to make informed decisions, they need to be provided with transparent and accurate information about finances, governance and overall cooperative performance.

Health Cooperative Financing

The following lessons are drawn from international experience, work in sub-Saharan Africa and Uganda's local experience [1, 12, 17, 19, 20]

1. Prepayment: Prepayment reduces administrative costs involved in running the scheme. Besides tracking all steps involved in care of patients, submitting claims requires a system of tracking and billing individual units of care, increasing the administrative requirements and investments by significant margins. Prepayment also provides an excellent way for providers to keep their cooperative members healthy, since lower treatment costs mean higher cost recovery and profit for the provider. Prepayment also overcomes the debt challenge that many providers face when patients paying out of pocket simply do not have the money to cover their treatment costs.
2. Provider dues: Providers are the primary financial beneficiaries of the cooperative scheme. As such, they have a responsibility to pay back into the scheme's reserve fund to ensure the scheme can continue to be well managed and well capitalized. The stronger and more well-run the cooperative, the more providers will profit from the partnership. In the model used by many cooperatives affiliated

with HealthPartners, providers are required to pay 10% of their annual surplus at the end of the year to ensure sufficient capital for scheme management the following year.

3. Member buy-in: While many members have little supplemental income with which to pay member dues, it has been noted that even minor financial contributions to the cooperative lead to improved member buy-in and reduced drop outs. For most cooperatives, membership dues per year are 1,000 UGX ($0.26 USD). Some cooperatives require member dues to be paid each time a member rejoins in the same year (assuming he/she dropped out for a time period) as a disincentive to drop out. Drop outs are a consistent challenge, particularly if a member does not fall ill in the first quarter of their membership because she sees little reason to remain in the scheme. At that point, member dues and communication about other member experiences are critical to ensure continued buy-in.
4. Copayments: Members are encouraged to seek early treatment for illness—that is one of the motivations of prepayment, to ensure those who need treatment seek it early so they remain healthier and the provider pays less to treat them. However, many healthy members are curious about services offered and may visit just to see what the provider has to offer. To reduce members seeking unnecessary care, cooperatives charge a copayment. It is a fairly nominal fee but it reduces visits by well members who use resources that could be otherwise invested in treating the sick.
5. No reinsurance: When risk is absorbed by another entity (i. e. an NGO or donor organization), providers are less likely to manage their scheme well—they may provide unnecessary treatments, laboratory services or medicines, fail to check identification, fail to collect premiums—since they know they have a fall back plan. If they don't make money, someone else will make it up for them. There is no incentive to properly manage a cooperative in this case. However, this lesson is applicable only in cases where members are capable of paying premiums, dues and copayments. In cases where potential members are too poor to even cover those costs, there is

some potential for government subsidies or cross subsidies (from more economically stable members) to cover the costs of the poor. But subsidies need to be carefully planned so as not to provide disincentive to providers to poorly manage their costs.

As is evident in the lessons listed above, HealthPartners has learned many of the same lessons found in the literature about what makes a CBHI successful. These lessons will be considered in 3.6 of this chapter to inform how Uganda can utilize these experiences to build a highly functioning community-based health insurance scheme.

Other LMICs Experiences with Health Cooperatives

There are many low and middle-income country (LMIC) experiences with CBHI from which Uganda can draw lessons to move forward with its own health sector development. We will take a brief look at the scheme structure, management and financing of some of the most applicable or most advanced LMIC cooperative and CBHI schemes to draw lessons:

China's Nation-Wide CBHI

The following lessons are a synthesis of experience and literature about CBHI in China [20, 21, 22, 23, 24, 25]. One of the largest examples of CBHI successfully implemented as a component of a larger national health insurance scheme is found in China. In 2002, China's central government made a commitment to expand health services in the rural sector as a means of reducing the gap in public services between rural and urban populations. In only ten years, the scheme has come to cover 98% of the total rural population (805 million people.) The rate of impoverishment due to health care costs has decreased and the use of health facilities has increased. Admittedly, China's political and financial structure allows for quick uptake of policies, since public funds immediately follow policy decisions, so some of the approaches China has taken will not be applicable to the Ugandan context. Additionally, while the scheme uses the term "cooperative" in its name, the relevance of the term is questionable, given its lack of member-driven democratic governance. Nevertheless, the rapid expansion of the scheme and its size make it worth briefly reviewing here.

Scheme Structure, Management and Funding

From the outset, China's highest decision-making authorities were committed to the cause of ensuring widespread rural coverage through what they called the Rural Cooperative Medical Scheme (RCMS). In 2002, the Central Committee of the Communist Party of China and the State Council put out a document entitled, "Decisions on the strengthening of the rural health system" which outlined the RCMS's sources of funding, level of fund pooling, benefit package and fund management.

The guiding principles came from the central government—outlined in the document referenced above—but the concrete implementation plans came from a combination of provincial and county governments. County-based offices manage funds and administration. Funds are pooled at the county level, with estimated populations of some half million people. The scheme is heavily subsidized—with 80% of funds coming from the government and only 20% from rural households. Initially, the benefit package offered was modest, with the focus on enrolling as many people as possible before expanding the package. Today, the package has expanded to include in- and out-patient services. Despite its name, China's RCMS lacks some of the critical tenets that define cooperatives – namely democratic governance, autonomy and independence. However, the following lessons are applicable to CBHI implementation:

1. Political commitment and building trust in the scheme are critical first steps.
2. Build on a formal health financing mechanism.
3. Prior to roll out of a national scheme, an implementation plan for how the CBHI will fit into the larger national health structure is needed.

4. Incentivize participation – In China, the central government matched local government investment to ensure subsidies for those who could not pay, reducing the schemes' vulnerability to adverse selection and increasing local investment.
5. Family-based enrollment, rather than individual, reduces adverse selection as well as increases rapid expansion.
6. Use media to spread the word about the scheme.
7. Quality of care is an ongoing challenge. China uses various indicators for paying providers, including patient satisfaction, rational use of drugs, and compliance with medical protocols.

Rwanda's Nation-Wide CBHI

The following lessons are drawn from relevant literature and experience in Rwanda [25, 26, 27, 28, 29, 30]. Rwanda is another LMIC that has rapidly implemented a CBHI scheme to cover majority of its population over the course of only a decade. Contextually, the experience of Rwanda is more comparable to that of Uganda. But, like China, Rwanda has seen uncommon political will and substantial government investment.

In 1996, user fees were reintroduced at health clinics, following dwindling donor support in the country. In response, utilization of health services fell and Rwandans were deprived of financial protection from high health care costs. In order to address these challenges, Rwanda piloted CBHI in 1999. The scheme, commonly known as 'mutuelles de santé' is now one of the largest CBHI schemes in sub-Saharan Africa, expanding health insurance coverage from 7% in 2003 to 84% by 2016/17. Utilization has increased, but some of that increase can be attributed to improvements the government has made to service availability, resources, and quality of care. Health care utilization has become more equitable and insured persons are more likely to use modern health care facilities. Being a CBHI member has substantially decreased out of pocket expenditures; as a result, the incidence of financial catastrophe owing to health care costs has dropped from 11% to 2% over a ten-year period.

Scheme Structure, Management and Funding

A critical element of Rwanda's CBHI structure is its linkages between each level of the health system. Pooled funding is coordinated at the district level, where each of 30 districts has a pooled risk fund. Each sector level health center has a CBHI branch and each village has a CBHI mobilization committee. Premiums are collected at the community level by the CBHI branch and are used to reimburse public health care providers. The scheme started out charging standard premiums and copayment rates. But by 2011, the scheme was adjusted to allow premiums to be paid on a sliding scale. The government pays full premiums and makes copayments for approximately 27% of the population that are too poor to pay for their own coverage and the rest pay based on their ability (72% pay approximately RWF 3,000 ($4.50 USD) per person per year and 1% pay 7,000 RWF ($10.50 USD) per person per year). Membership is family-based and compulsory for those who do not have other insurance. Rwanda's CBHI scheme is predominantly funded by member premiums (66%), followed by government (14%) and the Global Fund (10%). Copayments account for 6% of revenue and other insurance companies are mandated to provide the remaining percentage.

Summary of Lessons from Rwanda

1. Government support is key.
2. The Ministry of Health played a key role as policy initiator and champion.
3. Leadership at the national and local levels facilitated the rollout by developing and issuing relevant policies and laws.
4. The Ministry of Finance covers the premiums for the poor, so they can be included in the scheme.
5. The scheme is connected via a formalized health financing mechanism supported by the national government.
6. Rwandan values of mutual aid and solidarity assisted the rollout of the CBHI scheme.

7. Local leaders—particularly religious leaders—were relied upon to champion the scheme.
8. Rollout was assisted by donors, who facilitated pilot schemes and provided support and technical assistance through technical working groups organized and led by the MOH.
9. Media and government were leveraged to educate Rwandans about the importance of insurance.

Tanzania's Generic CBHI

The following lessons are a synthesis of literature and experience in Tanzania [8, 20, 30, 31, 32]. Until the 1990s, health care in Tanzania was paid for by the government. But health care reform in the 90s introduced cost sharing at government facilities, a national health insurance fund for civil servants and liberalization of private care facilities. A CBHI scheme (or 'mutual health scheme'), known as UMASIDA, was established in the late 90s with the support and technical assistance of the International Labour Organization (ILO) to address informal sector access to health care. This model is similar to the Ugandan cooperative model, with some significant departures in administration that have made it much less effective and sustainable.

Scheme Structure, Management and Funding

ILO worked with Tanzanian worker groups to launch the UMASIDA scheme. ILO defined the concepts and basic components and left each group to run its scheme as it sees fit. UMASIDA is largely managed by an apex organization which coordinates administration, training and technical assistance, as well as overseeing claims payments to providers. The relationship between the provider and the group is managed by group leaders who address member issues, control access to services, collect and adjust premiums as needed, and enforce rules. Premiums are paid by a group leader to the apex on a monthly basis, which reviews invoices for proper charges per agreements and pays out claims where applicable. The administrative burden of this payment system is considerable. Providers are contracted by UMASIDA and clinics have to comply with defined criteria like being able to perform certain laboratory tests and ability to provide primary care.

In general, the scheme requires prepayment of approximately Tanzania shs 1,500 ($1.30 USD) per month which covers a family with up to four children. Copayments of approximately Tshs 500 ($0.50 USD) are required at service locations to avoid overuse. This premium covers outpatient care, laboratory services and generic prescriptions. No costing method appears to have been used to determine the proper cost for the care required, so the scheme immediately ran into two problems that have continued to plague it: 1) insufficient funds to pay for care and 2) members immediately expected donor subsidies. UMASIDA has since raised prices multiple times, which has been poorly received by members and has led UMASIDA to the brink of bankruptcy. At its height, the scheme only covered a couple of thousand members.

Summary of Lessons from Tanzania

1. Do not implement a CBHI scheme with expectation of donor support. UMASIDA began with a donor mindset and was not able to move away from it.
2. Build the CBHI scheme with groups, rather than individuals, to avoid adverse selection.
3. Payments should be submitted in groups to leverage peer pressure and reduce drop outs.
4. Identification of those who have paid into the scheme from those who have not is critical to avoid free riders.
5. Communication of why premiums are rising is important. UMASIDA did not effectively communicate the reason for increased premiums and saw huge drop outs as a result.
6. Proper costing needs to be done prior to roll out to ensure that premiums will cover treatment costs.

7. Informal/unorganized health financing mechanism proved unsustainable.

Ghana's Nation-Wide CBHI

The following lessons are a synthesis of literature and experiences in Ghana [8, 20, 25, 33]. Structural adjustment policies in the mid-80s forced health care out of pocket payments to increase. CBHI had been a minor component of Ghanaian health care for half a century, but the high out of pocket costs provided additional incentive to implement CBHI on a wider scale. By 2002, CBHI schemes were seeing successes but coverage in the country was only 1-2%. In 2003, CBHI got a boost in support when Ghana rolled out its National Health Insurance (NHI) Act, which used mutual health organizations as a foundation for its structure. By 2010, 66.4% of the population was covered, almost half of which came from the informal sector. The unique aspect of Ghana's NHI is how it includes informal workers. It combines a network of CBHI entities with centralized authority and funding, which expands enrollment and improves sustainability.

Scheme Structure, Management and Funding

Under the National Health Insurance Act, Ghana organized district-wide insurance schemes. Every district is divided into Health Insurance Communities with each having their own Health Insurance Committees to oversee the collection of contributions and supervise their deposit into the District Health Insurance Fund. Every district also has a Health Insurance Assembly, which is the decision-making body responsible for creating their own constitution and guidelines for health insurance. The Assembly supports a board of trustees which hires a management team to oversee the daily work of the scheme.

Contributions to the scheme vary in accordance with district and ability to pay. Children, the elderly (over 70 years), pregnant mothers and the poor are exempt from paying into the health insurance fund. These exemptions account for 70% of NHI members. Others pay a range from 72,000 cedis ($5

USD) to 480,000 Ghana cedis ($33 USD) annually. Each district has its own identification system which enables residents to be categorized into a contribution payment category. Revenue from informal sector contributions accounts for only 3% of NHIS revenue. An additional 2.5% health insurance levy is paid by all Ghanaians on select goods and services to subsidize contributions and accounts for 74% of the NHIS revenue. A minimum package of benefits is dictated by the government and covers some 95% of diseases in Ghana, though districts can appeal to adjust their benefit packages. Once members have paid in full, they must wait six months to get health insurance identification card and facility attendance card. Then they are free to go to any public or private accredited health facility in Ghana in line with their benefit package. In the formal sector, 2.5% of workers' social security contributions (3% of NHI funding) is allocated to the National Health Insurance Fund and subsequently disbursed to the district schemes to cover formal workers' contributions. The system started out on a fee-for-service basis, but recognition that the model only incentivized over-diagnosis and over-prescription has led some to switch to capitation and diagnosis-related-group payments. Claims are managed by the National Health Insurance Authority, which processes 2.4 million claims each year. While the Ghana model has provided financial protection for the informal sector and improved health seeking behavior, it is not sustainable financially without government support given the low contributions of the informal sector and the high costs of claims management.

Summary of Lessons from Ghana

1. Fee for service claims payments are administratively cumbersome and provide perverse incentives to over-diagnose. Capitation is a more streamlined payment mechanism.
2. Generating substantial revenue from the informal sector is difficult. The addition of a health insurance levy was key to being able to finance the model, but depending on how it is levied, it may have a disproportionately negative impact on the poor.

3. Although contributions from the poor are supposed to be waived, evidence suggests that there is still significant inequity in the model. Policies need to be carefully crafted and applied to ensure the poor are covered.
4. Management capacity is still a challenge, in part due to its decentralization. Additional training is necessary to ensure proper management of the system in all districts.

Synthesis of Lessons Learned for Uganda and Other Countries Building Universal Health Care Schemes

By building on the strengths of CBHI schemes, particularly health cooperative schemes, and addressing their weaknesses through favorable policies and financial structures, Uganda can extend insurance coverage to informal populations not currently covered. Based on the lessons provided in this chapter and informed by previous literature as well as the experiences of Uganda and other LMICs, CBHI schemes have proven to be most successful when they are:

- Supported by significant political will,
- Financed by an organized health financing mechanism that leverages a large risk pool,
- Capably managed,
- Supported by laws and regulations that favor CBHI schemes, and
- Provided with sustained technical assistance.

The models examined in this chapter support the Wang and Pielemeier model of evolution. Those that have seen the greatest success in terms of population covered and financial sustainability have been those that have evolved from small and fragmented to nation-wide schemes. Success in these cases is not surprising, since these models have been able to generate large risk pools, professional management and financing. Those that have not evolved—like UMASIDA in Tanzania—more often than not succumb to the weaknesses of CBHI schemes. The HealthPartners cooperative experience has provided additional lessons, some of the most applicable are:

- Pre-payment or capitation--rather than fee for service claims--reduces the need for extensive administrative support and when properly costed, provides predictable funding sources for providers as well as incentive to reduce incidence of illness in the member population.
- Frame the CBHI/cooperative as a business that exists to meet the needs of its member-owners. Enforce member and provider buy-in, sense of ownership, self-responsibility and continually reassess the model to ensure it is meeting the needs of its member-owners.
- Enroll groups, not individuals, to expand the risk pool and reduce adverse selection
- Ensure identification is issued upon joining and always check identification before offering cooperative services to avoid free-riders.

These lessons are useful in helping craft a national scheme that covers the informal sector. But it should be acknowledged, as Wang and Pielemeier mention in their paper, that the transition from generic to nation-wide CBHI scheme can jeopardize some of the greatest benefits of the CBHI model, particularly its social benefits. Schemes that move from local ownership to national ownership reduce the ability of local communities to define their health care needs and meet them on their own terms. Local communities are no longer empowered. They cannot negotiate their own benefit packages or their own premiums. Stakeholders in these schemes--members and providers--may not reap the maximum benefit from the scheme, since risk and reward are both removed from them. Education and training are unnecessary, since management is concentrated at a higher level. Nation-wide models reduce local influence over provider quality and remove the relationship-building aspect of community-based health care.

Cooperative principles are particularly vulnerable in moving to a nation-wide CBHI scheme. Values like self-help and responsibility, equity and solidarity can be easily lost in the evolution. Whereas members in a cooperative scheme are considered owners and therefore contribute finances, time and skills, a large nation-wide scheme could make members 'beneficiaries' only--reducing their sense of ownership, their sense of self-help and their desire to contribute to the betterment of the community. Cooperatives also contribute to knowledge sharing and they empower their members, particularly women, to be leaders--both characteristics that have real impacts outside of the health cooperative. Stunting those outcomes could have consequences in terms of social and community development.

Assuming the social benefits of CBHI are valuable, could a CBHI scheme be developed that preserves the social benefits of cooperative schemes--like women's empowerment, education and training, and local leadership development--while creating a financially sustainable model? The answer is yes, but whether the Ugandan NHIS achieves this feat will depend on the details of how the scheme is planned and implemented.

HYPOTHETICAL SCHEME STRUCTURE, MANAGEMENT AND FUNDING

A scheme that preserved many of the social benefits of cooperatives would likely need to be spearheaded at the national level, with regulations in place that allowed the scheme to build a large risk pool (or pools) at regional or national levels by cross subsidizing to ensure financial sustainability [19, 24]. But decision-making would need to be left to democratically-elected Boards of Directors at the county or sub county levels, under overarching rules created by the national leadership about basic benefit packages, premium limits, basic provider services, and costing, etc.

Administrative functions like hiring staff, developing policies and procedures, setting premiums, enrolling members, establishing provider networks and payment protocols would all be done at the county or sub county levels. Communication with members and education about scheme performance would happen locally. Local BODs would host Annual General

Meetings where members address issues of premium costing, BOD elections, financial transparency, and scheme performance. Management would need to be drawn from and paid for by the membership, but professional training could be provided nationally to ensure adequate capacity. Partnerships and incentives with local universities to develop capable managers, as HealthPartners has recently done with International Health Sciences University, would accelerate and professionalize the process.

Membership would be voluntary with a strong recommendation that enrollment be family or group-based, rather than individual. Government could provide incentives for schemes to expand in the form of matching payments or tax deductions. Prepaid premiums, member and provider dues would be collected locally. Some percentage would need to be funneled to the county and national levels to ensure continued capital for operations and financial support for the nationalized risk pool, but much of the premium revenue should stay with providers locally to incentivize improved care, quality, and community development. An apex organization could be formed with members from the various county BODs to provide training, technical assistance and lobbying for favorable CBHI policies at the national level. This scheme would, of course, have to be fully supported by the government in order to build public trust in the market, create regulations that support the successful implementation, and provide financing. Marketing of the CBHI concept could be done both nationally and regionally. Regulations would have to be put in place to support the autonomy of CBHI schemes within the larger national scheme. Laws to protect democratic control, voluntary membership, and member economic participation as well as laws to promote equitable treatment of cooperatives and CBHI schemes, access to markets and due process would all need to be incorporated into a supportive regulatory framework.

Some level of financing would need to be provided for startup activities and to subsidize premiums for the poorest. Once the scheme is established, it may be able to provide its own cross subsidies--from the wealthier to the poorer and the healthy to the sick, though as seen in the LMIC examples above, no CBHI scheme is currently able to function well and go to scale without any government or donor financial support. Rwanda and Ghana, as in the case presented, as well as Senegal and Ethiopia, all incorporate some of these characteristics into their national health insurance schemes. Uganda would do well to study them more in depth before creating an implementation plan for a widespread CBHI model.

A national health insurance scheme that includes proven strategies presented in this chapter would accomplish the three outcomes originally outlined for an insurance model: 1) curb cost escalation, 2) improve the quality of care and 3) increase coverage. It would also preserve some of the most valuable characteristics of CBHI and health cooperatives like building trust, local empowerment and control, relationship-building between members and providers, knowledge sharing and member education.

Acknowledgments

This chapter is made possible by the generous support of the American people through the United States Agency for International Development (USAID). The contents are the responsibility of HealthPartners and do not necessarily reflect the views of USAID or the United States Government.

The editors are grateful to Proscovia Nnamulondo of Save for Health Uganda and Dr. Hizaamu Ramadhan of Uganda Management Institute for reviewing and enriching this chapter.

References

[1] HealthPartners. 2017. *Website*. www.healthpartners.com (Accessed 20th December 2017).

[2] Ghana National Health Insurance Authority. 2008. *National Health Insurance Authority Status Report: Operations*. Accra, GNHIA.

[3] Amzat, J. and O, Razum. 2017. *Towards a Sociology of Health Discourse in Africa. Switzerland*: Springer International Publishing.

Drechsler, D. and J, Jutting. 2007. Different countries, different needs: the role of private health insurance in developing countries. *Journal of Health Politics, Policy and Law*, 32(3), 497-534.

[4] Atim, C. 1998. *The Contribution of Mutual Health Organizations to Financing, Delivery, and Access to Health Care: Synthesis of Research in Nine West and Central African Countries*. Partnerships for Health Reform Project, Abt Associates Inc., Bethesda, MD.

[5] International Cooperative Alliance. 2017. *Website*: https://ica.coop/en/what-co-operative (Accessed on 20th December 2017).

[6] Carrin, G. 2003. *Community based health insurance schemes in developing countries: facts, problems and perspectives*. World Health Organization.

[7] Wang, H., N. Otoo, L, &Dsane-Selby. 2017. *Ghana National Health Insurance Scheme. World Bank Group*. Washington, DC.

[8] Zelelew, H. 2015. *Community Health Financing as a Pathway to Universal Health Coverage: Synthesis of Evidence from Ghana, Senegal, and Ethiopia*. Abt Associates. Bethesda, MD.

[9] De Allegri, M. R, Sauerborn, B, Kouyate, S, Flessa, S. 2009. Community health insurance in sub-Saharan Africa: what operational difficulties hamper its successful development? *Tropical Medicine and International Health;* 14(5), 586-596.

[10] Halvorson, G. 2007. *Health Care Co-Ops in Uganda: Effectively launching micro health groups in African villages*. Oakland, California, The Permanente Press.

[11] Agaba, G. and J, Mutanda. 2015. *Impact assessment of health cooperatives in southwestern Uganda*. Commissioned by HealthPartners.

[12] Uganda Bureau of Statistics. 2016. *Uganda Demographic and Health Survey: Key Indicators Report*. Kampala, UBOS.

[13] The World Bank. 2016. *The Uganda Poverty Assessment Report 2016*. Washington DC, The World Bank Group.

[14] Basaza, R. B, Criel, P, Van der Stuyft. (2007). Low enrolment in Ugandan Community Health Insurance Schemes: underlying causes and policy implications. *BMC Health Services Research*, 7(105).

[15] Hsiao, W. 2001. *Unmet Health Needs of two Billion: Is Community Financing a Solution*? HNP.

[16] Ministry of Health. 2019. *The Health Insurance Bill*. Kampala, Ministry of Health, Uganda.

[17] Ethiopian Health Insurance Agency. *2015. Evaluation of Community-Based Health Insurance Pilot Schemes in Ethiopia: Final Report*. Addis Ababa, Ethiopia.

[18] Uganda Community Based Health Financing Association. 2017. *UCBHFA Secretariat website*. (http://www.ucbhfa.org Accessed 1 October 2017).

[19] Jacobs, B. et al, 2008. Bridging community-based health insurance and social protection for health care-step in the direction of universal coverage? *Tropical Medicine and International Health Tropical Medicine and International Health*; 13 (2); 140-143.

[20] China Ministry of Health. 2009. *An analysis report on National Health Services Survey*. Beijing: Centre for Health Statistics and Information, Ministry of Health.

[21] Chinese Communist Party Central Committee and State Council. 2002. *Decisions on the strengthening of the rural health system* [Official Document No. 13]. Beijing: Chinese.

[22] Meng, Q. &Xu, K. 2014. *Progress and challenges of the rural cooperative medical scheme in China*. World Health Organization, Lessons from the field. http://www.who.int/bulletin/volumes/92/6/13-131532/en/.

[23] National Health and Family Planning Commission. 2013. *Statistical report on health and family planning development*. Beijing, China.

[24] Coheur, A; Jacquier, C., Diabate, V. Schremmer, J. 2007. Linkages between statutory social security schemes and community-based social protection mechanisms: A promising new approach, *World Social Security Forum*, Moscow, http://www.google.com/search?sourceid=navclient&ie=UTF-8&rlz=1T4SKPT_enUS449US449.

[25] East African Community. 2014. *Situational Analysis and Feasibility Study of Options for Harmonization of Social Health Protection*

System Towards Universal Health Coverage in the East African Community Partner States. Arusha, Tanzania: EAC, Secretariat.

[26] Iradukunda, AV. 2017. *Govt mulls raising Mutuelle de Sante fees*. Retrieved from http://www.newtimes.co.rw/section/read/208681/ (Accessed on 17th December 2017).

[27] Collins, D; Saya. and T, Kunda. 2016. *The impact of community-based health insurance on access to care and equity in Rwanda*. Management Sciences for Health, Medford, MA, USA.

[28] University of Rwanda and Management Sciences for Health. 2016. *The Development of Community-Based Health Insurance in Rwanda: Experiences and Lessons*. Technical Brief.

[29] McCord, M. 2000. *Micro-insurance: A case study of an example of the mutual model of microinsurance provision*. UMASIDA. Microsave.

[30] Kiwara, A. 2007. Group premiums in micro health insurance experiences from Tanzania. *East African Journal of Public Health*; 4 (1,), pp. 28-32.

[31] Dutta, A. 2015. *Prospects for Sustainable Health Financing in Tanzania: Baseline Report.* Washington, DC: Health Policy Project, Futures Group.

[32] Zelelew, H. 2015. *Community Health Financing as a Pathway to Universal Health Coverage: Synthesis of Evidence from Ghana, Senegal, and Ethiopia.* Abt Associates. Bethesda, MD.

[33] Ghana National Health Insurance Scheme. 2017. *Center for Health Market Innovations.* http://healthmarketinnovations.org/program/ghana-national-health-insurance-scheme (Accessed on 17th December 2017).

In: The Journey …
Editors: Robert Basaza et al.
ISBN: 978-1-53618-323-8

Chapter 5

NATIONAL HEALTH INSURANCE DEVELOPMENT IN UGANDA: THE STAKEHOLDER ENGAGEMENT, SLOW START ON THE THORNY, THIN PATH WITH MANY RIVERS, MOUNTAINS AND LIMITED VISIBILITY

Robert Basaza[1,2,*], Prossy K. Namyalo[3], Thomas S O'Connell[4] and David Ogubi[2]
[1]Gudie Incubation Centre, Kira Municipality, Uganda
[2]Uganda Christian University Mukono MPHL Program, Uganda
[3]Ndejje University, Faculty of Social Sceince,Uganda
[4]UNICEF, New York, US

* Corresponding Author's E-mail: rbasaza@gmail.com.

ABSTRACT

Uganda is the last East African country to adopt a National Health Insurance Scheme (NHIS). In order to lessen the inequitable burden of healthcare spending, health financing reform has focused on the establishment of national health insurance. The objective of this investigation was to depict how stakeholders and their power and interests have shaped the process of agenda setting and policy formulation for Uganda's proposed NHIS. The study provides a contextual analysis of the development of NHIS policy within the context of national policies and processes.

The methodology is a single case study of agenda setting and policy formulation related to the proposed NHIS in Uganda. It involves an analysis of the real-life context, the content of proposals, the process, and a retrospective stakeholder analysis in terms of policy development. Data collection comprised a literature review of published documents, technical reports, policy briefs, and memos obtained from Uganda's Ministry of Health and other unpublished sources. Formal discussions were also held with ministry staff involved in the design of the scheme and some members of the task force in order to obtain clarification, verify events, and gain additional information.

The process of developing the NHIS has been an incremental one, characterized by small-scale, gradual changes and repeated adjustments through various stakeholder engagements during the four phases of development: from 1995 to 1999; 2000 to 2005; 2006 to 2011 and 2011 to-date. In spite of political will and government buy-in, progress with the NHIS has been slow, more less like an unwinding river in mountainous gauge and is yet to be implemented. Stakeholders, notably the private sector, played an important role in influencing the pace of the development process and the currently proposed design of the scheme. This study underscores the importance of stakeholder analysis in major health reforms. Early use of stakeholder analysis combined with an ongoing review and revision of NHIS policy proposals during stakeholder discussions would be an effective strategy for avoiding potential pitfalls and obstacles in policy implementation. Given the private sector's influence on negotiations over health insurance design in Uganda, this paper also reviews the experiences of two countries with similar stakeholder dynamics.

ABBREVIATIONS

CHIS	Community health insurance scheme
HSSIP	Health sector strategic and investment plan
IRAU	Insurance regulatory authority of Uganda
MOFPED	Ministry of finance, planning and economic development
MOGLSD	Ministry of gender, labor and social development
MOH	Ministry of health
MOPS	Ministry of public service
NDP	National development plan
NGO	Non- government organization
NHIS	National health insurance scheme
NPA	National planning authority
NSSF	National social security fund
NTF	National task force
OOP	Out-of-pocket expenditure
PCHIS	Private commercial health insurance scheme
P4H	Providing for health
NRM	National resistance movement
SHI	Social health insurance.

INTRODUCTION

The East African report on social health insurance protection defines health insurance as a type of insurance against the risk of incurring medical expenses among individuals. An insurer has a pool of individuals, develops a routine finance structure and ensures that money is available to pay for the health care benefits specified [1] in the insurance agreement. The benefit is administered by a central organization such as a government agency, private business or not-for-profit entity [2].

This chapter underscores the lessons learnt over the last one and half decade with regard to the upcoming Ugandan national health insurance scheme. It builds on the previous research paper, "The players and the processes behind the National Health Insurance Scheme in Uganda. Notably, of the five East African countries, only Uganda is without a National Health Insurance Scheme (NHIS) [3]. Insurance can also overcome regressive aspects related to user fee policies [4, 5]. On both counts, Uganda is an anomaly. First, the drive for a health insurance policy has been sustained by the ruling National Resistance Movement (NRM), in power for over 30 years, and this has contributed to a strong sense of government ownership and deep institutional knowledge. Second, Uganda abolished formal user fees in 2001 in all public health units, (with the exception of private hospital wings) to eliminate financial access barriers [6]. Nonetheless, Ugandans have continued to experience high levels of Out-Of-Pocket (OOP) expenditure at 37% in 2014 down from 42% in 2013 [7] coupled with the indirect fees (such as transportation costs), supplementary fees to pay for medicines and supplies from private vendors, and illegal fees demanded by medical staff for purportedly free services [8]. Furthermore, the country has not respected some of the international treaties of which it ratified in the drive for universal health coverage (UHC). A good case is the 2001 Abuja declaration which called for at least 15% of their annual budgets towards health sector by 2015. It's only Rwanda in the East African region that has ever met this target [9]. The proposed Uganda NHIS is to be a contributory health financing mechanism, in which members pay a premium in exchange for a defined package of services, containing elements from both formal and informal employment sectors. The scheme shall be established by an act of parliament as part of proposed reforms to achieve universal health coverage. The NHIS has been promoted to mitigate regressive OOP spending and offer a more effective policy path for this country of 34.9 million people to have equitable access to universal healthcare [10].

Table 1. Key policies relevant to the proposed Uganda NHIS

Policy	Provisions relevant to NHIS
Constitution of Uganda 1995 [26]	• Objective XIV (b) is to ensure that Ugandans have access to health services • Objective XX is a commitment to take all measures to provide basic medical services to the population.
Health Sector Strategic Plan (HSSP) 2000/01–2004/05 [27]	• SHI as one of the key objectives of its healthcare financing component • Government would continue to develop and support alternative healthcare financing schemes.
Poverty Eradication Action Plan (PEAP) 2004/2005–2007/2008 [28]	• Objectives are pro-poor focused and are consistent with the MDGs • Human development and improving health outcomes among the key priorities.
Cabinet Minute No. 63 (CT 2006)	• Directed the Minister of Health to issue drafting instructions for the bill establishing the National Social Health Insurance Scheme to the First Parliamentary Council; Directorate in the Ministry for Justice responsible for legislative Drafting.
National Development Plan (NDP) 2010/11 – 2014/15 [29]	• Provides for the establishment of health-financing mechanisms (NHI and other community health-financing mechanisms) based on prepayment and financial risk pooling with the goal of achieving universal coverage and social health protection.
NRM Presidential Manifesto 2011–2016	• Provides for establishing a national health insurance scheme as one of the work programs in 2011–16.
Health Sector Strategic and Investment Plan (HSSIP) 2010/11–14/15 [30]	• Calls for health insurance, with the goal to increase financial access to healthcare and reduce the catastrophic expenses that impoverish households, to be introduced gradually, leading eventually to universal health coverage. • Commitment to fully harmonize health policies, Standards, and guidelines for the East African Community by 2014–15. • Guided by the principles of: (i) access for all to a minimum package of services; (ii) equitable distribution of services; and (iii) effective and efficient use of health resources
The second National Health Policy 2010 [14]	• Upholds the obligation of the government regarding citizens' access to healthcare • Guided by the same principles as HSSIP 2010/11–14/15
Cabinet Minute No. 84 (CT 2011)	• Directed the Minister of Health to issue additional principles of the bill to the First Parliamentary Council taking into consideration stakeholder concerns
Vision 2040	• The National Planning Authority of Uganda launched a long-term planning framework with a work program to develop a universal health insurance system through public private partner-ship as one of the mechanisms to transform the health sector.
Draft National Health Insurance Bill of 2014	• Ministry of Health submitted a revised bill to Ministry of Justice and obtained a new certificate of legislation compliance • Ministry of Health submitted this certified bill to Ministry for Finance and obtained a certificate of financial implications

Table 1. (Continued)

Policy	Provisions relevant to NHIS
National Health Insurance Bill 2020	• Ministry of Health tabled the bill in the Cabinet after obtaining a certificate of regulatory impact assessment from the Cabinet secretariat. It was passed in Cabinet and thereafter tabled the bill in the Parliament. It is currently before the Health Committee of Parliament.
The East African Community Social Health Protection Report 2014	The East African Situation Study of Options for harmonization of Social Health Protection Systems Towards Universal Health Coverage in the East African countries points out that Uganda continues to stand alone as the only East African country without a social health insurance scheme which could affect harmonization of social health protection mechanisms in the region.
The National Development Plan 2015/16-2019/20	• Underlines the plan by government to work towards achieving Universal Health Coverage (UHC) through establishing a national health insurance scheme while harnessing synergies from public private partnerships and strengthening the referral system. • Seeks to establish a national health insurance scheme as a revenue generation mechanism in health financing.
Health Financing Strategy 2015/16 – 2024/25	Underlines that the poor and vulnerable population groups are to be protected from hardships as a result of out-of-pocket payment for healthcare through introduction of social health insurance scheme and increasing government general revenue funding for health care.
NRM Presidential Manifesto 2016-2021 Tabling and seeking approval by the cabinet June 2019 Tabling NHIS Bill in Parliament Aug 2019	• Aims at introduction the Universal Health Insurance Scheme as one of the work programs in the health sector. Cabinet approved the bill. Hon. MOH tables the bill in the Parliament and still pending before the Health Committee Parliament.

The first part of the chapter provides the following: a process analysis of the four phases of health insurance development and contextualized stakeholder management. The second part is a stakeholder analysis that covers the following: (i) a description of the methods used for the stakeholder analysis; (ii) a categorization of the key policy players; (iii) a discussion of the process of stakeholder engagement and management strategies employed by the government; and (iv) a conclusion with lessons relevant to policy makers on how a stakeholder-driven and broadly inclusive policy development process can increase the likelihood of policy implementation. With no elaborate social health protection mechanism currently in place and soaring OOP health costs, the development of an equitable, sustainable health-financing mechanism for the NHIS is seen as a key strategy to achieve the MDGs [11], and now sustainable development goals (SDG). Table 1 summarizes the key government policies to reduce poverty and improve health and their relevance to the evolution of the current version of the proposed NHIS.

THE PROCESS OF NHIS DEVELOPMENT

The development of the NHIS has taken place in four phases: Phase I, from 1995 to 1999; Phase II, from 2000 to 2005, Phase III, from 2006 to 2011, and Phase IV, from 2012-to date. These phases are based upon key events linked to the health sector and the national 5-year planning frameworks.

Phase I, 1995–99: 'People's Power'

This period was characterized by decentralization, the introduction of user fees, and CHI schemes, and we label this as 'people's power'. During this period, people made an effort to engage in decisions that governed their lives. The period saw the introduction of health-financing reforms and broad decentralization. Subsequently, there was passage of the 1997 Local Government's Act and there after decentralized governance and delivery of health services. In 1996, Uganda's Ministry of Health (MOH) commissioned the first feasibility study on health insurance, and some limited CHI pilot schemes were attempted [12]. The feasibility study was exploratory and looked at the potential for establishing social health insurance in Uganda. The study pointed out the limited knowledge that existed in Uganda with regard to social health insurance policies and administration. It recommended a further detailed examination of implementation arrangements [12]. The first Poverty Eradication Action Plan, which was finalized in 1997, established a participatory national development strategy based upon pro-poor and poverty-reduction policies, including pro-poor budget allocation [13]. These policies led to the first National Health Policy (1999–2009); its objectives included universal coverage to achieve improved health outcomes and equity, and it was financed through a countrywide Social Health Insurance (SHI) model [14]. Subsequently, the government launched the Health Sector Strategic Plan 2000–05, which increased spending on health, coupled with higher user fees and was introduced in 1993 as a precondition for a World Bank loan [15]. Shortly after, a presidential order in March 2001 abolished user fees, having been driven by both a 1999 World Bank report on the regressive impact of user fees on healthcare access and the desire to bolster re-election chances in the upcoming 2001 presidential elections [15, 16]. The years 1997 to 2001 represent a period during which differences of opinion among the key internal stakeholders within the MOH on the proposed SHI model intensified [12]. Moat and Abelson pointed out that the 'big man', the president, abolished user fees without due consultation among key stakeholders and clients, including civil society, the managers of public health facilities, and private providers [17].

Phase II, 2001–05: 'Hopeful Start'

This was a phase of SHI design that we describe as a 'hopeful start'. Continued poor financing of health-system access led the government to commission a second feasibility study on health insurance. This aimed to align the design of health insurance with the first health policy, the Health Sector Strategic Plan of 2000–05, and to provide insight into implementation plans [18]. Specific recommendations included phased SHI implementation starting with the formal sector; with time, this would expand to informal-sector protection [19]. The result was the establishment in 2005 of the SHI Secretariat by the MOH. A cabinet paper was produced by this secretariat in 2006, 'Principles of SHI,' were circulated to stakeholders, including other government ministries, professional medical associations, trade unions, and local government associations for sensitization and consultation [20]. The

MOH also undertook visits to Thailand, India, and Tanzania to study models of national insurance, and conducted additional studies with Providing for Health (P4H), an alliance of four European governments (Germany, Switzerland, Spain, and France); two multilateral organizations (the World Bank and African Development Bank); and two United Nations agencies (International Labor Organization -ILO and the World Health Organization-WHO), among others. Following a 2- year consultative process, the updated principles of SHI were presented to the cabinet and adopted in 2006 [20]. The Minister of Health was directed to prepare a bill on establishing SHI and initiate a legislative process for introducing SHI.

Phase III, 2006–10: 'Stakeholder Concerns'

We categorize this period as 'stakeholder concerns'. Following resistance to the bill to establish SHI, the MOH set up a multi-sectoral working group, the National Task Force (NTF) to spearhead a participatory design process for drafting a revised insurance bill. An attempted stakeholder analysis was undertaken to help identify issues relevant to the design of the health insurance scheme. However, the analysis had minimal utility since there was an apparent lack of experience on the part of the working group in carrying out and using stakeholder analysis for policy development. Furthermore, this attempt at stakeholder participation was not genuinely broad based. The National Social Security Fund (NSSF) did not join the health insurance scheme despite an appeal by the NTF for it to do so [21]. One factor was that such stakeholders as the NSSF perceived health insurance to be a project of the MOH rather than a broad-based government initiative [22]. The NTF produced a revised SHI bill in 2008 as well as a framework of its organizational aspects and the accreditation of providers.

Though the NTF succeeded in bringing together public and private sectors in a common forum, it did not effectively create ownership among the private-sector players or engage in a redesign of the proposed scheme. Instead, the NTF sought to prioritize the sensitization and buy-in of stakeholders by advocating for the existing SHI framework [21]. As a result, the proposed SHI plan still lacked the backing of some major stakeholders—notably private-sector employers and employees. In early 2009, the NTF held workshops for the cabinet and parliament, which prompted the government to request technical support from P4H. The P4H assessment identified low levels of stakeholder involvement as an impediment to implementing SHI, and it recommended that their engagement be significantly reinforced [21]. The assessment also recommended greater inter-ministerial coordination as well as openness, clarity, and public engagement with respect to the SHI and—importantly—to its alternatives. Interviews with stakeholders from the NTF revealed that the majority of the task force members supported the general idea of SHI, but they felt that the plan lacked clarity with regard to efficiency, effectiveness, and supervision. The NTF stakeholders also questioned the equity of a phased SHI implementation according to employment group [21, 23].

The recommendations of P4H and other development partners led in October 2009 to the prime minister creating a cabinet sub-committee composed of four state ministers: health; finance planning and economic development; public service; and labor. The drafting committee was expanded to include public- and private-sector experts, such as the Insurance Regulatory Authority of Uganda, private insurers, and representatives of CHI schemes, so as to broaden the ownership and buy-in.

In 2010, a review by the MOH and WHO explored feasible health-financing options for health insurance. By mid-2011, the cabinet sub-committee redrafted the SHI principles. It started by successfully negotiating a name change from an SHI plan, which implied that it alone could potentially cover all citizens, to an NHIS, which signaled the use of multiple insurance component plans to cover various segments of the population. This was strongly endorsed by private insurance providers, which were concerned about market displacement because it preserved their existing market of private-sector firms [24]. The sub-committee also secured a consensus on establishing a solidarity fund with tariffs and rates for healthcare, greater market liberalization for the provision of health insurance, and adding a CHI component to cover individuals working in the informal sector. The private sector was reassured that its commercial health insurance schemes and third-party health administrators would not face competition from the NHIS because the SHI component was limited to targeting public-sector workers and the CHI pertained to the informal sector. Though direct presidential endorsement was not provided, the cabinet approved these revised principles in September 2011, with the expectation that the NHIS scheme would be introduced in 2013 [25].

Phase IV, 2011 to 2020: 'The Rivers, Mountains and Limited Visibility'

Undoubtedly, Uganda is enriched with sound policies although their implementation remains a challenge. Firstly, the NRM manifesto for the period 2011-2016 on health insurance seemed a good gesture but ended up without a concrete deal for Ugandans. Secondly, the HSSIP 2010/11-2014/15 drafted clear strategies and targets which included allocating more resources to the preventive services and functions in the strategic period with substantial evidence that they were indeed more cost effective compared to the curative functions, simply ended as a blue print [26]. In the same boat, the Ministry of Health got entangled in an uphill fight when it presented the revised draft bill to the Ministry for finance seeking a certificate of financial implications to facilitate the tabling of the bill in Cabinet and Parliament in 2014. The Ministry of Finance wrote several letters seeking clarification from Ministry of Health and subsequently a certificate of financial implication was issued in 2016. The design of the universal national health insurance has remained a key issue in the long-term country planning frameworks: Vision 20/40, the second National Development Plan 2015/16-2019/40, the Health Sector Development Plan 2015/16-2019/20 and the NRM Presidential Manifesto 2016-2021. In the same period, the later part of 2015 saw the policy championed behind the NHIS process depart from the Ministry of Health for personal engagements [27]. Communication from the Task Force on the design of the scheme indicates that currently, the schemes are being redesigned to ensure a stepwise approach starting with civil servants alone and the informal sector to come on board later- 5 years after the launch of the scheme. The entire process is more like a winding river in mountainous gauge in an environment with limited visibility. In 2018, the Honorable Minister of Health submitted the bill to Cabinet, passed in 2019 and now before the Health Committee of Parliament. The delay in Cabinet was the new requirement of a regulatory impact assessment of any bill before being tabled in Cabinet. Regulatory Impact Analysis (RIA) is a systemic approach to critically assessing the positive and negative effects of proposed and existing regulations and non-regulatory alternatives.

Financing the Proposed NHIS

The NHI scheme can improve overall health financing if it 'raises adequate funds for health, in ways that ensure people can use needed services, and are protected from financial catastrophe or impoverishment associated with having to pay for them' [28]. Diverse sources of healthcare funding are often cited as useful for achieving a stable health financing system [29], and a mixed financing approach is common in Africa [30, 31]. It was proposed that the planned NHIS be financed by 4% of payroll deductions from employees with an additional 4% from employers [32]. The plan calls for a solidarity fund, into which annual contributions from the government, donors and the formal sector will pay a portion of their premium to cover indigent (including unemployed) persons—currently estimated at 19.7% of the population [33]. Formal-sector workers and up to four of their dependents—accounting for approximately 10% of the country's population—will be eligible to join the Social Health Insurance Scheme and Private Commercial Health Insurance Schemes at the inception of the NHIS.

The informal-sector workers and their dependents will join the Community Health Insurance Scheme, and in this way the NHIS will progressively cover the entire population. The above percentage contributions were calculated in a feasibility study by Harvard University and Makerere University Schools of Public Health in 2001 [19] and in 2008 by the WHO/MOH using SimIns (health insurance software).

Table 2. Relationship of NHIS[*], community health insurance scheme and private commercial health insurance scheme

Common arrangements	**NHIS**	**CHIS[*]**	**PCHIS[*]**
Role of proposed Board of Directors of NHIS	For oversight of health insurance schemes and in-house operations of public sector workers and their dependents' scheme, the social health insurance scheme	Represented on the Board. The NHIS Board will provide regulations	Represented on the Board. The NHIS Board will provide regulations
Regulation by Insurance Regulatory Authority of Uganda.	Yes	No	Yes
Participation in solidarity funds	Provides funds to CHI for indigents	Membership for indigents shall be paid by the NHIS	Contributes part of the premium to the solidarity fund for paying premiums to indigents
Specific issues			
Ownership	Government	Private	Private
Current coverage	-	5–10% of the population where the schemes exist	1% of the national population
Target membership	Public formal-sector workers and their dependents	Informal-sector workers and their dependents.	Employees and dependents from the private formal sector
Proposed/current source of funding	Mandatory payroll deductions and contributions from both employees and the government	Contributions from personal earning for those above the poverty line. Payment from the solidarity fund for those below the poverty line	Mandatory payroll deductions and contributions from employees and private-sector employers
Benefit package	Stipulated in the bill	Negotiated with the private healthcare providers	Negotiated with employers, trade unions, and individual members and insurance companies.

The NHIS will initially generate 153.183 billion shillings in 2013, gradually increasing to 675.552 billion shillings by 2018 (2012 exchange rate: 2,500 shillings per 1 US$). The scheme will initially enroll public formal-sector employees and their dependents and generate more money as enrolment rises among both the informal and formal private sectors workers and their dependents. Virtually all in-patient and out-patient care provided within Uganda will be covered by NHIS. Further details of the benefit package are provided for in a schedule in the NHIS bill [18]. The mechanisms for coping with the envisioned increase in patient load in accredited health units and expansion of services in the underserved areas once the scheme begins have yet to be worked out. Table 2 summarizes the current components of the proposed NHIS. The objective of this chapter is to present the path of development of the National Health Insurance Scheme in Uganda, the key role of stakeholders' engagement and the unwinding path to establish the scheme. Various terms are used to describe the entities involved, such as actors, players, stakeholders, and interested parties [34]. We use the term 'stakeholder' to signify an 'entity with a declared or conceivable interest or stake in a policy concern' [35]. This includes individuals, organizations, collectives, and various groups, either formally organized or unorganized. This process of managing stakeholders is a vital factor for achieving health policy change [36, 37].

METHODS

The methodology adopted here is a single case study of agenda setting and policy formulation related to the proposed NHIS in Uganda. It involves an analysis of real-life context, the content of proposals and the process, and a retrospective stakeholder analysis using the single instance of NHIS policy development.

Table 3. Partial list of key stakeholders shaping Uganda's NHIS by group affiliation

National government actors	Public sector	Private sector	Civil society	Donors
(i) Parliament (ruling party and opposition)	(i) National Social Security Fund (NSSF)	(i) Private for profit and non-profit providers	(i) NGOs	(i) Providing for Health (P4H)
(ii) President (executive president)	(ii) Insurance Regulatory Authority of Uganda (IRAU)	(ii) Private insurance companies	(ii) Trade unions and employee groups	(ii) Swedish Development Agency
(iii) Prime minister	(iii) National Planning Authority (NPA)	(iii) Private-sector foundation	(iii) Health professional associations	(iii) UK Department of International Development
(iv) Cabinet		(iv) Uganda Manufacturers Association		(iv) Belgian Technical Cooperation
(v) Ministry of Health		(v) Community health insurance schemes		
(vi) Ministry of Finance, Planning and Economic Development (vii) Ministry of Public Service (viii) Ministry of Gender, Labour and Social Development (ix) Local governments (district and urban authorities)		(vi) Federation of Uganda Employers		

The choice of research methods matched our goal of providing a retrospective analysis of the participants (both individuals and groups) engaged in the NHIS development. We also examined how action or inaction by the stakeholders influenced this process, and investigated the context in which the process unfolded. Data collection was carried out through literature reviews of published and unpublished documents; these included technical reports, policy briefs, and memos obtained from the MOH plus an analysis of secondary data collected by UNICEF for a survey of NHI in 52 countries [30]. Formal discussions with selected senior health ministry staff and NTF members involved in the design of the scheme were conducted to obtain clarifications, verify events, and obtain background information. Express permission to carry out this research and access to all data was granted by the MOH. This study was part of the work program of the Ugandan health sector approved by the government, donors, and all stakeholders as indicated in the second National Health Policy and Health Sector Strategic and Investment plans.

Stakeholder Analysis and Design of the NHIS

Although political stability is important [38], the successful design and implementation of health insurance also greatly depends on consensus among the key stakeholders and securing their support for all its elements, including the benefits package, level of contributions, and details of who contributes what proportion of the premiums [39]. The process of stakeholder analysis refers to a methodology for 'systematically gathering and analyzing qualitative information to determine whose interests should be taken into account when developing and/or implementing a policy or program' [34]. Stakeholder analysis allows policy makers to anticipate the challenges and the relative ease with which the policy can be introduced and understand how to manage the process more effectively. Effective engagement of stakeholders also ensures the sustainability of a reform because it provokes 'the creation of actors who will defend their new interests in the political process' [40].

Stakeholders and Their Policy Positions

The development of the NHIS involved numerous sectors and stakeholders. For example, the MOH identified 55 stakeholders that have in some way shaped the CHI—one of the four component schemes of the NHIS [55]. Our analysis focused on selected stakeholders at the core of the overall NHIS design process (Table 3).

Stakeholders Offering a High Degree of Support and Having High-Level Influence

Support of the NHIS by the government was high at both ministerial and cabinet levels. The following provided ongoing support for the NHIS, most notably during the second and third phase of its development: the MOH; Ministry of Finance, Planning and Economic Development; Ministry of Gender, Labor and Social Development; and Ministry of Public Service. Their support was formally expressed through a cabinet minute ('decree') in September 2011. Parliament has viewed the NHIS as a means to improve access to quality services and alleviate the suffering of the Ugandan population. A parliamentary sub-committee in April 2012 gave the go-ahead to the NTF to finalize drafting of the NHIS bill for final approval. Two cabinet decrees (2006 and 2011) and the Ruling Party Presidential Manifesto calling for NHI signaled strong support at the cabinet level. The Prime Minister, who chairs the cabinet, made a public statement, expressing his support for the NHIS. Even members of the opposition party voiced their support [32]. As of late 2011, the various political actors remained united behind the NHIS as an all-party achievement. However, the president has not publicly backed the latest NHIS plan. This may signal the awareness of the executive branch that some stakeholders, such as private-sector insurers, still harbor concerns that the NHIS could negatively affect growth of the private insurance market. P4H worked through the MOH to provide technical support for the NHIS design process as well as implement criteria and strategies. Through P4H, the World Bank participated in the NTF. The bank catalyzed stakeholders' engagement, such as by funding a study tour to three East Asian countries (Thailand, Vietnam, and China) so that cabinet members could examine SHI schemes. The WHO country office also participated in the NTF to advise on design issues and support sensitization of parliament and cabinet members. One critical area of WHO support was for a combined team from the ministries of health and finance to develop robust estimates for NHIS revenue and expenditure using SimIns software [21].

Stakeholders Offering a High Degree of Support and Having Medium-Level Influence

As an agency with vested power to determine priority areas for national development planning, the National Planning Authority (NPA) produced the National Development Plan 2010/11–2014/5, wherein establishing an NHIS was set forth as a core area of health sector reform [29]. The second National Development Plan 2015/16 – 2019/20 spells out NHIS as one of the health sector interventions that will lead to attainment of Universal Health Coverage (56). As a member of cabinet, the NPA chairperson also provided strong support for the NHIS. The Insurance Regulatory Authority of Uganda (IRAU), which oversees all insurance operations in the country including health insurance, was an important stakeholder in influencing the NHIS design and planned implementation. As a member of the NTF, the IRAU played a key role in drafting the cabinet memo on NHIS principles that was approved in 2011.

Stakeholders Offering a High Degree of Support and Having Low-Level Influence

CHI schemes are managed by private organizations, which have only limited influence on proposed government reform, though their support for NHIS was strong. For them, the NHIS represented an opportunity for growth and expanded enrolment in CHI schemes. The CHI schemes influenced policy through their umbrella network, the Uganda Community-Based Health Financing Association, which lacks formal opportunities for influencing NHIS policy beyond membership of the NTF.

Stakeholders Offering a High Degree of Support and Having Medium-Level Influence

As an agency with vested power to determine priority areas for national development planning, the National Planning Authority (NPA) produced the National Development Plan 2010/11–2014/5, wherein establishing an NHIS was set forth as a core area of health sector reform [41]. As a member of cabinet, the NPA chairperson also provided strong support for the NHIS. The Insurance Regulatory Authority of Uganda (IRAU), which oversees all insurance operations in the country including health insurance, was an important stakeholder in influencing the NHIS design and planned implementation. As a member of the NTF, the IRAU played a key role in drafting the cabinet memo on NHIS principles that was approved in 2011.

Stakeholders Offering a High Degree of Support and Having Low-Level Influence

CHI schemes are managed by private organizations, which have only limited influence on proposed government reform, though their support for NHIS was strong. For them, the NHIS represented an opportunity for growth and expanded enrolment in CHI schemes. The CHI schemes influenced policy through their umbrella network, the Uganda Community-Based Health Financing Association, which lacks formal opportunities for influencing NHIS policy beyond membership of the NTF.

Stakeholders Offering Medium-Level Support and Having a High Degree of Influence

The private sector, including the Uganda Manufacturers Association and Private Sector Foundation, wields substantial influence. This is largely through the Presidential Investment Forum, in which the private sector advises the president on market development, employment, and taxation policy. However, the proposed SHI bill generated strong negative reactions from non-MOH stakeholders, primarily in the private sector, who believed that SHI would displace private health insurance schemes [40]. Employers, specifically manufacturers, were concerned that the obligation to pay a share of the insurance premium for enrolled employees would increase production costs [42]. Formal sector employees and employers were apprehensive about the capacity of the government to manage the SHI Fund: this was the result of a history of public funds mismanagement [12, 42], most notably cases involving the Global Alliance for Vaccines and Immunization and the National Social Security Fund [43, 44]. In addition, concerns were raised about a potential worsening of the already poor quality services because the costs to meet increased demand for services would exceed the additional resources forecasted to be generated by SHI [23].

Subsequent to concerns raised by several influential stakeholders, the president halted the process and called for more dialogue between the MOH and the private sector. Key actors in the health sector thought that this was simply a health-sector issue and did not adopt a multi-sectoral approach and engagement among all stakeholders. The MOH and NTF were able to garner some support from the private sector by negotiation. Although some concerns remain in the private sector, for example about NHIS increasing production costs and the risk of business failure, the position of the NHIS is now closer to that of a supporting coalition than it was during the second phase of its development. A second influential group is that of private insurers, who are concerned about losing their market share to the NHIS [45]. A recent study showed that only 36% of surveyed employers would continue subscribing to private health insurance schemes after implementation of the NHIS [12]. Responding to their interests rather than the position they took on NHIS, the MOH has agreed on a strategy of liberalizing the health insurance industry. The trade unions have special seats in the national parliament, which allow them to participate in policy debates. Trade unions are concerned about the proposed 4% payroll deduction from workers' pay [42]. However, discussions are continuing with the unions and the NSSF about whether the 4% can be part of the NSSF contribution made by employees. It should be noted that some large employers would fully cover the 8% contribution because of existing collective bargaining agreements mandating health insurance coverage.

Stakeholders Offering Medium-Level Support and Having Medium-Level Influence

Local governments wanted the scheme to be implemented. However, they had strong concerns over the potential burdens that would be imposed in terms of administration as well as the level of their contributions to its financing [46].

Stakeholders Offering Medium-Level Support and Having Low-Level Influence

Health professional associations, such as the Uganda Medical Association and the Nurses and Midwives Association, questioned whether the NHIS could have the intended impact of increased access to quality care and improved population welfare [47]. Although the media could potentially play an influential role by raised public awareness of the NHIS, the main media outlets had neither adopted a position about establishing the NHIS nor focused much coverage on the proposed health reform legislation.

Stakeholders Offering a High Degree of Opposition

During Phase I, the management of the NSSF was also opposed to the establishment of a SHI scheme. That NSSF management felt that it was the best-qualified institution to run a SHI scheme [48], and it viewed the creation of an SHI as threatening its authority and influence.

RESULTS AND DISCUSSION

Health Financing

Households contribute over 40% of Total Health Expenditure funds, which results in great inequalities in general health and access and use of healthcare services because it disproportionately constrains poorer people from accessing the necessary care. This situation also increases the incidence of catastrophic expenditure, thereby increasing the level of poverty [49]. Current health-financing trends provide the option of a pooled mechanism for health insurance in the case of limited government funding.

Stakeholder Engagement

Roberts et al. proposed that to create alliances for supporting new policies and introducing health reform, it is necessary to develop political strategies to manage the power and positions of stakeholders. Some political strategies seek to change the position of stakeholders; some aim for redistribution of power among the stakeholders; some pursue a change in the number of players or their group affiliations; and some seek to change the perception of the problem or the solution [37]. The private sector was vehemently opposed to the establishment of virtually any NHI arrangement until the Minister of State responsible for health insurance addressed them in a collective forum during Phase II. Negotiations were conducted in the presence of a neutral arbitrator from the World Bank. Among the grievances of private-sector stakeholders were their exclusion from NHIS planning consultations, the possibility of increases in the cost of production, and lack of representation at the planning level [42]. The private sector demanded a voice in selecting NTF members and being guaranteed participation in NHIS design and management [45]. In addition, the private sector desired liberalization of the scheme's operations. The negotiations led to a more comprehensive NTF that represented all stakeholders, with provisions for liberalizing the insurance plan then being adopted in a new NHIS draft bill.

The private-sector representatives attended NTF meetings and carried out sensitization missions for other stakeholders. Similarly, private commercial insurers were concerned about business being lost to the NHIS, and they maintained a strong involvement in the NHIS design process. The previous management of the NSSF, which was also opposed to the NHIS, was replaced. The new management adopted the view that a comprehensive insurance scheme was desirable, and it demonstrated its commitment by agreeing to sit on the NTF. Civil society groups did not take on a strong position on the NHIS and remained largely passive, possibly through a lack of awareness of the significance and implications of the NHIS for the general public. Furthermore, non-state providers of services were more concerned about ensuring sufficient financing to maintain existing services than examining ways to expand those services. Some concerns such as those related to the impact on fair access to quality healthcare were shared among stakeholders with different levels of support and influence. NGOs and donors were both concerned whether the NHIS could deliver on its promise of better quality and more equitable healthcare [47]. The change of position of such stakeholders as the NSSF and private insurers illustrate the key characteristics of stakeholders on how support for a policy can shift over time, and in this case such shifts provided opportunities for developing NHIS policy.

Additional Considerations

The stability of the Ugandan political system, with the president in office for over 30 years, offers a strong advantage for the NHIS. Recent health reform success cases (like in Bangladesh, Kyrgyzstan, and Ethiopia) emphasize the importance of strong bureaucracies and a stable political system for effective implementation of such reforms [38]. Conversely, the impetus for the NHIS was strongly associated with democratic reforms in Uganda, in which the NRM won multi-party elections in 2006, 2011 and again in 2016. This is similar to the cases of Ghana and Tanzania, where health insurance was included in the election manifesto of the ruling party and introduced both to meet the expressed wishes of the electorate and ensure a presidential legacy [4 &50].

The role of the presidency in Uganda can be compared to that of Kenya during the development of the National Social Health Insurance Fund (NSHIF) law [51, 52]. An inter-sectoral taskforce was established to prepare a national strategy and legislation as a first step towards formulating the NSHIF. In 2004, the Kenyan parliament passed the NSHIF bill, but the president did not accede to it, partly because he had not been fully consulted on the bill [53]. There was also a stalemate where the Ministry for Health and Ministry for Finance did not agree on implementation modalities of the then designed Kenyan scheme. This clearly indicates the relevance of stakeholder analysis and engagement at the highest level; Uganda and other countries could learn from this experience.

Conclusion

Uganda provides an interesting case study for exploring how planning for NHI has evolved since 1995 and moved to the current stalemate. The design of the NHIS was characterized by small-scale, gradual changes and adjustments during all three phases of development. Despite willingness by some sections of government, resistance by various stakeholders played an important role in constraining the pace of the development process as well as in shaping the design of the proposed NHIS.

The study points out how a policy-making process characterized by negotiation, bargaining, and adjustment of policy actions responded to stakeholders' aspirations and positions. Among other ways, the stakeholders influenced the policy makers in changing the design and name of the proposed health-financing reform from SHI to NHI. Stakeholders were also influential in changing the design from a single to multiple schemes and in the immediate incorporation of the informal sector in the early design and operation of the scheme.

In line with its neighbors, Uganda set out to establish an NHIS to provide for more equitable access to services as well as for a more durably financed health sector. The initial proposal received a low level of support, mainly because the plan was developed without taking into consideration key stakeholders and thus failed to meet their concerns. The preparation and planning for NHI in Uganda was overly concerned with policy content, and very little thought was given to stakeholder engagement. Even the study tours to three East Asian countries failed to identify the general process by which policy reform was negotiated, stakeholders analyzed, and political institutions engaged and managed. The initial phase had a limited knowledge base and minimal available research to provide guidance and practical examples for the political economy in establishing NHI. Lacking a good evidence base, the sponsors of the NHIS relied largely on technical solutions and past experience with other health reforms.

The case of the NHIS in Uganda thus offers several valuable lessons:

(i) It is vital to undertake a comprehensive stakeholder analysis as part of any substantive health-sector reform to identify, address, and overcome concerns before they harden into inflexible opposition. An intensive, detailed stakeholder analysis during the design process could pinpoint rising issues or threats minimize, obstacles to passage, build coalitions, and channel information and resources to promote and sustain reform implementation [35, 37].

(ii) The positions of stakeholders can be influenced to shape the direction in which they develop over time. Thus, policy makers and implementers need to consider periodic re-categorization of stakeholders to capture emerging positions and shifting power dynamics as well as sustain their continued engagement. If stakeholder analysis is not reevaluated at regular intervals, it can slow down or halt the policy design and development process—even when there is strong support from senior executive and legislative representatives.

(iii) The private sector represents an important stakeholder in health-financing reforms, and its role needs to be carefully considered. Comprehensive feasibility and actuarial studies of the health insurance scheme need to be complemented by broader political economy analyses and social impact assessments that specifically examine the potential effects of SHI on employment and investment in the private sector.

(iv) A situational analysis of health-sector policies and recent health reforms may need to be conducted to identify potential conflicts with the proposed NHI plan. Launched after major political change and against the backdrop of abolition of user fees, the NHIS faces additional challenges that overlap with technical issues, stakeholder management, and the common apprehension that often surrounds major health reforms. It is necessary to address these challenges. This will entail reconciling the views of two different sets of stakeholders on how to overcome the financial barriers to access: those advocating user fee abolition to achieve universal healthcare; and those advocating the imposition of some level of contribution for insurance coverage as the vehicle for universal healthcare. For example, Kenya and Tanzania had to reintroduce user fees before implementing their NHI schemes [50, 52, 54]. The government of Uganda may need to re-evaluate the impact on changes in the level of community financing of services in the current environment of abolishing user fees before pressing on with stakeholder discussions and NHIS implementation [5, 52].

(v) A growing body of literature supports the argument that an analysis of stakeholders and the policy arena is highly relevant to health-policy reform and represents an important first step in developing plans for NHI. This chapter points out how policy making is a complex process with an unstable and rapidly changing context. The use of stakeholder analysis in predicting and managing the future is time limited, and it is desirable that it be supplemented by other policy analysis approaches, such as the Delphi method [55]. Our results from this Uganda case study add to the body of evidence and offer useful information to policy makers and those tasked with designing and implementing SHI in low- and middle-income countries or similar settings.

We recommend further research to elucidate additional details on the related technical, substantive, and operational factors. This would clarify the major reasons for preventing an NHI scheme from being established in Uganda as compared with the East African countries that have advanced further in this area. Such studies could provide greater information on the enabling and constraining factors, such as the scope of services included in insurance benefit packages, the level of private contributions, and the level of coverage provided to various sub-populations, particularly the poor, informal-sector workers, and other groups not covered by private insurance plans.

REFERENCES

[1] East African Community. (2014). *Situational analysis and Feasibility Study of Options for harmonization of Social Health Protection systems towards Universal Health Coverage in the East African Community Partner States*, Arusha: East African Community.

[2] Basaza, R., O'Connell, S. T. & Chapcakova, I. (2013). Players and processes behind the national health insurance: a case study of Uganda. *BMC Health Services Research*, pp. 13-357.

[3] Bainemigisha, H. (2011). *Your Rights*, vol. XIII, pp. 8–9. Kampala: The Uganda Human Rights Commission; pg 8–9.

[4] Rajkotia, Y. (2017). *The political development of the Ghanaian National Health Insurance System: lessons in health governance*. Bethesda, MD: Health Systems 20/20 Project, Abt Associates Inc.

[5] Witter, S. (2010). *Mapping user fees for health care in high-mortality countries: evidence from a recent survey*. London, UK: HLSP Institute.

[6] Basaza, R. K., Criel, B. & Van der Stuyft, P. (2010). Community health insurance amidst abolition of user fees in Uganda: the view from policy makers and health service managers. *BMC Health Serv Res*, *10*, 33. doi:10.1186/1472-6963-10-33.

[7] Ministry of Health. (2015a). *Annual Health Sector Performance Report 2014/15*, Kampala: MOH: Government of Uganda.

[8] Pariyo, G., et al. (2009). Changes in utilization of health services among poor and rural residents in Uganda: are reforms benefitting the poor? *Int J Equity Health*, *8*, 10.1186/1475-9276-8-39.

[9] Organization of African Unity: *Abuja declaration on HIV/AIDS, tuberculosis, and other related infectious diseases* (OAU/SPS/ABUJA/3). http://www.un.org/ ga/aids/pdf/ abuja_declaration.pdf.

[10] Uganda Bureau of Statistics. (2014). *National Housing and Population Census 2014*, Kampala: UBOS: Government of Uganda.

[11] Kalk, A., Groos, N., Karasi, J. C. & Girrbach, E. (2010). Health systems strengthening through insurance subsidies: the GFATM experience in Rwanda. *Trop Med Int Health*, *15*, 94–9.

[12] Zikusooka, C. M. & Kyomuhangi, R. (2008). EQUINET Discussion Paper. In *Private medical pre-payment and insurance schemes in Uganda: What can the proposed SHI policy learn from them*? Edited by Loewenson R. Southern Africa: Harare: Health Economics Unit, University of Cape Town in the Regional Network for Equity in Health in East and Southern Africa (EQUINET).

[13] World Bank: *Uganda country brief.* http://go.worldbank.org/ 8XKQR04V10.

[14] Ministry of Health. (1999). *National Health Policy*. Kampala: MOH, Government of Uganda.

[15] Okuonzi, S. A. (2004). Learning from failed health reform in Uganda. *Br Med J*, *329*, 1173–1175.

[16] Deininger, K. & Mpuga, P. (2004). *Economic and welfare effects of the abolition of health user fees: evidence from Uganda*. Uganda: World Bank policy research working paper.

[17] Moat, K. A. & Abelson, J. (2011). Analyzing the influence of institutions on health policy development in Uganda: A case study of the decision to abolish user fees. *Afr Health Sci*, *11*, 578–586.

[18] Basaza, R. (2012). *Personal discussion with Dr Francis Runumi*, Head of Planning Ministry of Health edition.

[19] Berman, P., et al. (2001). *A feasibility analysis of social health insurance in Uganda. Uganda*: Harvard School of Public Health.

[20] Government of Uganda. (2006). *Cabinet Minute No. 63 (CT 2006)*. Kampala: Government of Uganda.

[21] Providing for Health. (2010). *Health Financing Reform & Social Health Protection*, *Specifying the options*; Follow up visit and dialogue between Ugandan Stakeholders and a P4H Team. Providing for Health. Uganda: Republic of Uganda.

[22] Ministry of Health. (2007). *Proceedings of the Task Force meeting*. Kampala: MOH, Government of Uganda.

[23] Orem, J. & Zikusooka, C. (2010). Health financing reform in Uganda: how equitable is the proposed National Health Insurance scheme? *Int J Equity Health*, *9*, 23.

[24] Government of Uganda. (2011). *Cabinet Minute No. 84 (CT 2011)*. Kampala: Government of Uganda.

[25] Nabatanzi, V. (2011). Uganda: *Government to Start Health Insurance Scheme*. In The New Vision. Kampala: All Africa Global Media.

[26] Ministry of Health. (2010). *Health Sector Strategic and Investment Plan 2010/11-2014/15*. Kampala: MOH, Government of Uganda.

[27] Basaza, R. (2015). *The NHIS in Uganda* [Interview] (21 October 2015).

[28] World Health Organization. (2007). *Everybody's business: Strengthening health systems to improve health outcomes: WHO's framework for action.*, pp. 56. Geneva, Switzerland: WHO.

[29] Cichon, M. & Normand, C. (1994). Between Beveridge and Bismarck: options for health care financing in Central and Eastern Europe. *World Health Forum, 15*, 323–328.

[30] Charlet, D., Chapcakova, I. & O'Connell, T. (2012). *UNICEF survey of National Health Insurance in 52 countries in Africa and Asia, with an emphasis on Social Health Insurance*: Phase 2 survey results. New York: UNICEF.

[31] O'Connell, T. S. (2012). *National health insurance in Asia and Africa: Advancing equitable Social Health Protection to achieve universal health coverage*. New York: Programme Division, UNICEF.

[32] Ministry of Health. (2019). *National Health Insurance Bill*. Kampala: MOH, Government of Uganda.

[33] World Bank: *Uganda country brief*. http://go.worldbank.org/8XKQR04V10.

[34] Schmeer, K. (1999). *Stakeholder analysis guidelines. In Policy toolkit for strengthening health sector reform*. Bethesda, MD: Partnerships for Health Reform, Abt Associates Inc.

[35] World Bank: *Stakeholder analysis*. http://go.worldbank.org/40BSM5Z9B0.

[36] Walt, G. & Gilson, L. (1994). Reforming the health sector in developing countries: the central role of policy analysis. *Health Policy Plan, 9*, 353–370.

[37] Roberts, M. J., Hsiao, W., Berman, P. & Reich, M. R. (2008). *Political analysis and strategies. In Getting Health Reform Right: A Guide to Improve Performance and Equity*. New York: Oxford University Press, Inc.

[38] Balabanova, D., McKee, M. & Mills, A. *'Good health at low cost' 25 years on: what makes a successful health system?* London: London School of Public Hygiene and Tropical Medicine.

[39] Gottret, P. & Schieber, G. (2006). *Health financing revisited*: A practitioner's guide. Washington DC: The World Bank.

[40] Berman, P. A. & Bossert, T. J. (2000). *A decade of health sector reform in developing countries: what have we learned?* A paper prepared for the DDM Symposium. Washington, D.C.: Data for Decision Making Project, International Health Systems Group, Harvard School of Public Health.

[41] National Planning Authority Uganda. (2011). *National Development Plan 2010/11-2014/15*. Kampala: National Planning Authority, Uganda.

[42] Barya, J. J. (2011). Uganda. *In Social security and social protection in the East African community*. 1st edition. Kampala: Fountain Publishers; pg 27-44.

[43] GAVI Secretariat. (2008). *Doc # AF.14 - report on Uganda ISS*. In GAVI Alliance and Fund Board meeting, vol. 2012. Uganda: GAVI.

[44] Tsekpo, A. & Hudson, A. (2007). *Parliamentary strengthening and the Paris Principles: Uganda case study*., pp. 12–14. London: Overseas Development Institute; 2009:12–14.

[45] World Bank: *Assessment of the proposed Uganda mandatory health insurance scheme*, October 8 – 12, 2007: Final Report. Kampala: World Bank.

[46] Ministry of Health. (2012). *Reports on sensitization of Social Services Committee of Parliament and stakeholders*, 2011–2012. Kampala: MOH, Government of Uganda.

[47] Ministry of Health. (2008). *Sensitization on the proposed National Health Insurance Scheme report*. Kampala: MOH, Government of Uganda.

[48] Jamwa David, C. (2009). *National Social Security Fund: To be, or not to be? An analysis of the clear case for NSSF's continued role in securing the social security of the workers of Uganda*: report. Uganda: Uganda National Social Security Fund.

[49] Xu, K., Evans, D. B. & Aguilar-Rivera, A. (2005). *Designing Health Financing Systems to Reduce Catastrophic Health Expenditure*. Technical Briefs for Policy-Makers.

[50] Humba, E. (2011). *Pioneering social health insurance in Tanzania: the case of the National Health Insurance Fund (NHIF)*. In MMS

Bulletine, vol. Improving Access through Effective Health Financing – Reader of the Swiss Tropical and Public Health Institute's Spring Symposium 2011. Basel, Switzerland: Network Health for All, 55-62.

[51] Ngilu, C. K. (2004). *We have to make health the engine for economic development. In Social Health Insurance – Systems of Solidarity: Experiences from German development cooperation.*, pp. 17. Eschborn, Germany: Deutsche Gesellschaft für Technische Zusammenarbeit (GTZ) GmbH.

[52] Carrin, G., et al. (2007). 2007. Health financing reform in Kenya – assessing the social health insurance proposal. *S Afr Med J*, *97*, 130–135.

[53] Chuma, J. & Okungu, V. (2011). Viewing the Kenyan health system through an equity lens: implications for universal coverage. *Int J Equity Health*, *10*.

[54] Gilson, L. (1996). *The lessons of user fee experience in Africa.* Johannesburg, South Africa: EDI Health Policy Seminar.

[55] Brugha, R. & Varvasovszky, Z. (2000). Stakeholder analysis: a review. *Health Policy Plan*, *15*, 239–246.

[56] National Planning Authority Uganda. (2015). *National Development Plan 2015/16-2019/20.* Kampala: National Planning Authority, Uganda.

In: The Journey …
Editors: Robert Basaza et al.
ISBN: 978-1-53618-323-8

Chapter 6

THE CONTRIBUTION OF PRIVATE COMMERCIAL HEALTH INSURANCE TO UNIVERSAL COVERAGE IN UGANDA; A BUMPY DITCHED ROAD WITH MULTIPLE CHALLENGES AND OUTPUTS

Prossy K. Namyalo[1,*], Karen Nansubuga[2,3], Sam Atuhura[4], Angela N. Kawooya[5,6], Dan Musiime[7] and Robert Basaza[8]

[1]Ndejje University, Faculty of Socail Sceinces, Uganda
[2]International Air Ambulance, Uganda
[3]The World Bank Washington, US
[4]Clarity Consulting, Uganda
[5]International Health Sciences University, Uganda
[6]Bugema University, Uganda
[7]Jubilee Insurance Company, Uganda
[8]Gudie Incubation Centre, Kira Municipality, Uganda and Uganda Christian University, MPHL Program

---

[*] Corresponding Author's E-mail: pnkiddu@gmail.com.

ABSTRACT

Introduction

Uganda since 2006, has been in the process of drafting a National Health Insurance Scheme Act. At the beginning of drafting the process, Private Commercial Health Insurance (PCHI) was one of the components and was later dropped in the current May 2019 edition of the bill. Persons that are not in formal employment and they don't want to join community health insurance will be enrolled in the PCHI.

Methods

The methodology used is descriptive and included reviewing of records from a number of institutions including Uganda Insurers Association, Insurance Regulatory Authority, Health Maintenance Organizations (HMOs), Association among others. Records were supplemented with literature on PCHI in Uganda and other countries, and the authors used both published and grey literature.

Findings and Discussion

Majority of the PCHI are employer-based schemes and 75% of the schemes have their own facilities, with the remaining schemes run by insurance companies. These schemes target private formal sector workers and their dependents. Very few members join as individual families. The formal sector is easy to enroll in and can afford relatively higher premiums compared to the rural informal sector workers. There were nine (9) paid up HMOs with a gross written premium (GWP) of UGX 52,159,269,966 in 2016. Currently there are 7 Health Insurance Organizations registered by the Insurance Regulatory Authority. The HIOs operate with a more open access network of providers and generally charge higher premiums than the HMOs. Their costs are likely to be higher since they do not own their own facilities. In the past, insurance services were considered to be a luxury as it was assumed that only the rich people could afford the high premiums. This led to low penetration levels in country. Besides, due to high poverty levels, private health insurance is not well consumed. Private health insurance by nature is costly and only a certain proportion of the population may afford it. Depending on how many lives an insurer has on the schemes, extrapolating these figures to total cost shows that this is not a profit driven market because of the high loss ratios. The challenges and lessons learnt are explained in this chapter. In addition, the chapter presents three case studies on specific companies in the business of PCHI.

ABBREVIATIONS

AAR	African Air Rescue;
GWP	Gross Written Premium;
HIO	Health Insurance Organization;
HMO	Health Maintenance Organization;
IAA	Internal Air Ambulance;
NHIS	National Health Insurance Scheme;
PCHI	Private Commercial Health Insurance;
UGX	Uganda Shillings.

INTRODUCTION

Basic healthcare is one of those needs that one would think is a necessity and that it should be available to the population either at no cost or if it is at a cost, then it should be affordable. In a number of developed countries, the governments have taken tremendous steps towards providing healthcare at no cost to its population. This is proving to be an uphill climb for low income countries. In the UK for example, the government provides for healthcare through the NHIS, in the US, although there is private health insurance, the government has different plans like the Medicare and Medical Aid. The US passed the Affordable Healthcare Act in a bid to make healthcare affordable to its population and so other governments have carefully planned for health care access to their populations to make it affordable and equitable. This story changes when it comes to developing countries where healthcare is characterized by escalating health care costs, poor health care infrastructure, inadequate tax revenues and unsustainable donor funds which has a huge effect on household incomes. Inevitably masses are forced to pay out of pocket for their healthcare expenditure [1-4].

Developmental organizations have in recent years put emphasis on social health insurance as a means of reducing healthcare cost burden on the populations with the hope of making healthcare more accessible financially and achieving universal health coverage. Social health insurance consists majorly of compulsory contributions into a health fund basket in return for packaged benefits in the hope to decrease out of pocket expenditures and increase access and equitable distribution of health resources. Contributions from households and enterprises are usually based on income while government contributions are based on taxes [5, 6]. Despite the efforts, very few countries have registered success in this area. Rwanda and Ghana are some of the countries in Africa that have registered success in social health insurance, with Rwanda having more than 90% of the population covered under health insurance schemes and Ghana at 45% coverage [7-12].

Uganda has no contributory social health insurance scheme and its budget allocation to health services in the financial year 2018/2019 was at 7.4%. This allocation is still far below the 2001 Abuja Declaration and the 2003 Maputo Declaration, both of which recommended funding to the health sector of up to 15% of their respective national budgets. The cost of health services in Uganda has continuously risen over the past years making the allocation insufficient to cater for the crippling health sector where the government has and is still struggling to provide for such a critical public service [13-15]. Private expenditure which includes out-of-pocket payments, donor financing that flows through non-governmental organizations and prepaid plans account for three-quarters of health financing in Uganda. However, like in most low-income countries, private prepaid plans made a negligible contribution to health financing [7, 14-16].

Private voluntary health insurance represents small risk-pools in form of small and highly fragmented community-based and commercial health insurance schemes. Community-based schemes in Uganda are communal, facility and third managed and have problems with financial, social and technical sustainability [17-21]. Private Health Insurance schemes are still in their infancy and cover less than 2% of the population who are based in key urban areas (especially Kampala). They are usually provided by corporate employers for their employees and dependents. Whereas private insurance schemes are mainly located in urban areas, the community-based schemes are in rural areas [14, 16, 22].

The country has since 2006 been in the process of drafting a National Health Insurance Scheme bill. At the beginning of drafting the process, Private Commercial Health Insurance (PCHI) was one of the components and was later dropped in the current May 2019 edition of the bill. Persons that are not in formal employment and don't want to join community health insurance will be enrolled in the PCHI [14, 23]. However, in a situation where the masses have a choice to join or not to join the PCHI. Whereas poverty levels and the cost of insurance for many Ugandans remain high, it would not be a question of if or not to join, but rather an inevitable decision not to join the schemes. The poor people cannot afford the premiums [16, 24].

METHODOLOGY

The methodology used is descriptive and include reviewing of records from a number of institutions including Uganda Insurers Association, Insurance Regulatory Authority, Health Maintenance Organizations (HMOs) and Health Insurance Association among others. Records were supplemented with literature on PCHI in Uganda and other countries. The authors used both published and grey literature.

FINDINGS AND DISCUSSION

The History of Private Commercial and Other Private Informal Health Insurance Schemes in Uganda

The history of private commercial and other private informal health insurance schemes is well documented in the East African report on social health protection. The first scheme, African Air Rescue (AAR) was started in 1994. The majority are employer-based schemes and 75% of them have their own facilities, with the remaining schemes run by insurance companies. These schemes target private formal sector workers and their dependents. Very few members join as individual families. The formal sector is easy to enroll and can afford relatively higher premiums compared to the rural informal sector workers. They enroll children over three months, exclude the elderly (over 65 years of age unless previously enrolled) and cover about 1% of the population mainly in urban areas. They face major challenges like lack of tariffs and rates in Ugandan health care systems (providers charge the amount they want), weak regulation and poor quality of care. The quality of care for both scheme and non- scheme patients is the same. Patients are only identified at the point of payment [7, 25]. The country has informal community health insurers like funeral groups which also lend money for health care and transportation of the sick like "Engozi". They are localized, small in scale and voluntary. Furthermore, there is family assistance where family members contribute money for health care for the sick. Like all small homogenous entities, they are unable to diversify risk across the population and are susceptible to adverse selection [26, 27].

The Current State of Private Health Insurance

Private commercial Health Insurance in Uganda is composed of 2 main streams; the Health Maintenance Organizations (HMO) and Health Insurance Companies (HICs) [28].

Health Maintenance Organisations

Health Maintenance Organizations (HMOs) or Health Membership Organizations for the case of Uganda are membership organizations that provide pre-paid medical schemes to their members. They usually own facilities where members can go and access services at no extra cost other than the premiums charged. Members are usually charged reasonable premiums for a combination of health benefits [25]. The first HMO registered in Uganda was African Air Rescue (AAR) in 1994. There were nine (9) paid up HMOs with a gross written premium (GWP) UGX 52,159,269,966 in 2016. International Air Ambulance (IAA) dominated the market share with 46%, followed by African Air Rescue (AAR) Health Services (43.30%) and Case Medical care (5.45%) in the third position. Others are: International Health Network, Kadic Health Foundation, Nakasero Healthcare, International Medical Link, St Catherine Clinic and Lisa Medical Centre. The GWP presents 11% growth from 2015. The HMOs accounted for 8% up from 7.7% in 2015 of the gross premium underwritten by the insurance industry which increased from UGX 612 billion in 2015 to UGXs 634 billion in 2016. This represents 3.6% growth [28]. By nature, HMOs provide mainly primary and secondary level care with a few providing tertiary level care. They have defined benefit packages that are offered to their members. Premiums are dependent on the kind of package the individual or corporation wishes to take up. In total, the HMO's had 10 members as at the beginning of 2017. Majority of the members are under group policies that are taken by employers for their employees and their eligible dependents. A few individuals sign up on their own under the individual policies although these would normally pay higher premiums. They majorly operate within the country with very few offering packages that cover regional expenses. Premiums range from as low as Ugandan Shillings (UGX) 350,000 to as high as 700,000 per person per annum [25, 28].

Health Insurance Organisations

Health Insurance Organizations (HIOs) are fully licensed insurance companies with a health and life insurance portfolio. There are 7 HIO's registered by the Insurance regulatory authority. These are: Jubilee Insurance, UAP, Sanlam, Liberty Health, Insurance Company of East Africa, First Insurance and APA. The HIOs operate with a more open access network of providers and generally charge higher premiums than the HMOs. Their costs are likely to be higher since they do not own their own facilities [28-30]. There is no systematic study on the health insurance premiums of HIO because they are entwined, and are part of overall insurance premiums of the companies. However, about two years ago, IRA started reporting on medical insurance premiums separately from other lines of business.

Despite players having been providing health insurance for more than 23 years, a regulatory framework was recently concluded. The Insurance Act 2011 provides for the regulation of medical insurance including private commercial health insurance schemes which includes HMOs and HIO. Figures from the regulatory authority indicate a 43% growth in premiums written for medical insurance between 2013 and 2014 [17, 31]. During the period 2015/2016, the Medical Insurance portfolio was registered at UGX 56 billion with a retention rate of 61%. Insurance penetration in Uganda is still below 1%, which is the lowest in Africa. Out of a population of more than 36.4 million people, only 1% is enrolled on private commercial health schemes who are mainly supported by formal employment [28, 30-34]. The biggest numbers of people enrolled in private medical insurance are in group policies with employers procuring the service either for their employees only, or for the employees and their dependents. Premiums are charged differently from one insurer to another. Some premiums are charged as a flat fee and for some, it's charged based on age bundles as a risk factor. In other cases, premiums are charged based on the underwritten risk. However, variations in health insurance premiums and health care packages which are caused by underwriting have to a greater extent been considered unacceptable on ethical grounds [5, 28, 31].

Worth noting is that due to market demands and increased competition, benefit packages have evolved to include both out-patient care and In-patient care as the core benefits. Extra benefits like dental and maternity, wellness cover and regional cover serve as enhancers. It is no longer about risk only for insurance in its true sense should cover elective procedures, pre-existing and chronic conditions. There are different kinds of insurance that is offered-depending on the preference of the client and also the amount of risk the provider is willing to take on. Some clients have insurance that gives the entire risk to the insurance company [29, 31, 35].

There are also clients that prefer to have the insurer manage their finance pool for healthcare as a third party. This means the client is taking care of the entire risk and not the insurer. However, the insurer charges a fee for administering the scheme. This is what MINET (formerly AON) does in all its operation areas. The third option which is usually adapted by corporations with large numbers of beneficiaries is a hybrid of the two kinds where the client gives the insurer a portion of the risk and the rest of the risk stays with the client. Depending on what the client needs, the premiums will differ depending on what kind of risk is involved. Similarly, it should be noted that some corporations' entities have a direct relationship with health facilities with the later billing those companies directly thereby avoiding the administrative fees that are typically charged by insurance companies [36 - 39].

Impact on Accessibility of Healthcare Services

In a country like Uganda, most insurers use the same service providers especially upcountry where service provision levels are still lacking. Kampala being the business hub in Uganda and also the capital city houses the highest number of hospitals and clinics. Insurers use government facilities especially the private sections of these facilities in addition to the private not for profit providers and the private hospitals and clinics [40,41]. Since the insurer has an obligation to meet the clients' need for healthcare services, they are put in a position where they create a demand for services to be available to the client. This has translated into an increase in the number of private hospitals and clinics in the country. Entrepreneurs and investors view insurance as a stable source of income and profit. They start clinics with the hope that they will be signed by the insurers and therefore increase their cash flow and hopefully profit [30, 31, 34, 35].

HMOs are forced to set up more healthcare facilities which give the population easier access in terms of distance and quality of services due to demand from their clients and competition from the other insurers. A case in point is AAR and IAA where AAR has increased the number of clinics owned by the HMO to a total of 10 clinics in 2015. IAA's sister company IMC has moved from 1 clinic on Kampala Road in 2000 to 13 in 2017 found in the different areas of the country. Given their nature, such providers create a benchmark for quality healthcare in the places they exist [25, 31, 41, 42]. In most cases, they will be run by qualified personnel with clear quality management systems in place. The level of services they provide is higher than their counterparts because they are driven by profit and competition. Nonetheless, the service offered has to give value for money to the client. For other providers, there is almost no choice other than improving their services so as to attract more private insured clients. Some insurers also run capacity building programs with these providers as corporate social responsibility initiatives. The competition created by insurance companies drives key factors of service accessibility and quality for the healthcare providers [35, 36, 40, 41]. It's important to note that more employers are increasingly taking medical insurance of their staff members seriously because it directly impacts on the productivity of the company in terms of increased morale and improved health state.

Impact on Out of Pocket Expenditure and Household Income

Uganda's current health financing accounts for 17.8% of the current health expenditure which translates to US$10 as against the recommended minimum public health financing target of $84 [14, 21]. Even when the country has made considerable progress in reducing the poverty levels from 54.4% in 1993 to the current 27% [24], the population living below the poverty line is still big. This leaves the population in a dilemma with expenditures including expenses for health. With no financial risk protection policies or measures, the services are highly dependent on the ability to pay and not the need which does not help the country's health indicators in terms of mortality and morbidity rates. With over 36.4 million people, Uganda has the lowest penetration of Insurance in the East African region which is noted at less than 2% [7, 14, 21, 24, 33]. This leaves the bigger percentage of the population struggling with huge out-of-pocket payments for their health due to the absence of a national health insurance scheme. The out-of-pocket expenditures are at 40%, pushing a big population to suffering catastrophic health expenditure [15, 21, 24].

The continuous declining state of public health services has in a way pushed the demand of private health services which are looked at, as a positive indicator because this growth comes with improved services in terms of quality and accessibility. Yet, because the health centers are run as businesses, access to the services come at a cost, and in some centers, the cost of service is very high. Besides the small percentage of Ugandans on health insurance schemes, health expenditure is known to have devastating impact on household incomes and poverty levels. In fact, a number of households have been left with no income or savings due to huge health expenditures [15, 21, 38, 41]. For a country with a heavy burden of disease, small tax base (where public facilities are characterized with high drug stock outs), there is almost no option for an average Ugandan than out of pocket expenditure [14, 43]. Out of pocket payments are a very inequitable mechanism because they create an undeniably huge burden on households and also generate obstacles for access of services for the poor. This is even worse since in most cases health care cost cannot be determined earlier. This makes it quite difficult to plan for [15, 21, 24, 40].

Challenges Faced by PCHIs

Medical Insurance is not like any other kind of insurance, because it deals directly with life; claims are experienced from the first day of signing off. And with little or no regulation especially in the past, competition and the unregulated market-insurers have found themselves dealing with quite a number of challenges.

In the past, insurance services were considered to be a luxury as it was assumed that it was only the rich people that could afford the high premiums. This led to low penetration levels in country. Worse still, due to high poverty levels, private health insurance is not well consumed. Private health insurance by nature is costly and only certain percentages of the population may afford it. Although this is changing with premiums being as low as UGX 350,000, not many individuals can still afford it and yet it's these same low premiums that are no longer sustainable for the insurers because of the rising cost of doing business. Statistics show an average cost per an outpatient visit of approximately UGX 90,000 and an annual average number of visits per person at 5. Depending on how many lives an insurer has on the schemes, extrapolating these figures to total cost shows that this is not a profit driven market because of high loss ratios. Worth noting is that outpatient visits account for more than 70% of insurers' claim spend/out-go [24, 25, 28, 31, 42]. Ugandan experiences with PCHI schemes are elaborated in case studies below

Case Study 6.1: Former Micro-Care Insurance Company

Micro-care insurance company is being presented as a case of poor control of health insurance services that existed in Uganda [34, 35, 37]. Most players struggle with sustainability challenges due to high claim ratios, stiff and unhealthy competition leading to undercutting of prices and un-realistic underwriting processes which have caused players to exit the market. The sector witnessed the closure of Microcare, one of the biggest players in the market in 2009. Microcare was started as a community-based financing scheme in 2000 that turned into a private firm in 2004. Over the years, due to the low premiums charged and un-healthy underwriting practices the firm experienced growth of over 200% through the years until 2007. However, during this time, the company had poor fraud control structures and was grappling with high claims. In 2009, the company filed a case with the high court seeking to wind up business. It was reported that Microcare had failed to clear medical bills with different service providers amounting to over 2billion shillings. Relatedly, just more recently in August 2015, the insurance regulatory authority also de-licensed another member (African Premier Health (APH) due to the same reasons. This and other factors like the lack of knowledge by the public on insurance principles and fraudulent practices on the part of the providers and the members themselves makes it harder for the market to grow as desired. Worth to note is that around 2011, the East African Underwriters withdrew their flagship medical products from the market because of the immense losses they were making [31, 37, 38, 40].

Case 6.2: HMO - International Air ambulance

International Air ambulance (IAA) a health maintenance/membership organization in Uganda was inaugurated in 2001 as part of IAA Healthcare. It is part of the International Medical Group. Other International Medical Group companies are International Hospital Kampala (IHK), International Medical Centre (IMC), IMG Pharmaceuticals (IMGP) and the International Medical Foundation (IMF). IAA's schemes are serviced primarily through IMG facilities therefore insuring flexibility, higher limits and quality services. There are IMG 12 health units, and other close to 40 health units in Kampala and 99 countrywide. IAA Healthcare also works with 180 other health service providers countrywide ensuring that wherever clients are, they will be able to access services. IAA Healthcare was recognized as a leading health insurance provider by the Private Sector Foundation Uganda in 2014 [28, 29, 42].

Case 6.3: Jubilee Insurance Company

Jubilee Insurance Company of Uganda Limited was first licensed to offer medical insurance services in Uganda in 2007 by the Insurance Regulatory Authority (then known as Uganda Insurance Commission). Jubilee had already been offering medical insurance in Nairobi where it is headquartered. Jubilee Uganda saw this as an opportunity to extend much needed services to its clientele in Uganda while at the same time expanding its product offering hence income. Jubilee's medical portfolio quickly grew from a business of UGX 353M in 2007 to UGX 35billion in 2016. Currently Jubilee Insurance is the largest HIO in Uganda. By 31 March 2018, Jubilee had insured 60,000 lives and this number is growing. Jubilee has partnered with more than 200 service providers across the country where its clients can seek medical services [21, 44].

REFERENCES

[1] Shi, L. and D. Singh. 2013. *Essentials of the U.S. health care system* (3rd ed.). Sudbury: Jones and Bartlett.

[2] World Health Organization (WHO). 2013. *Health Systems Financing: The Path to Universal Health Coverage: Plan for Action.* Geneva: WHO.

[3] Leive, A. and K. E. Xu. 2008. Coping with out-of-pocket health payments: empirical evidence from 15 African countries. *Bulletin of the World Health Organization* 86 (11): pp 849–856.

[4] Gottret, P. E. and G. Schieber. 2006. *Health financing revisited: a practitioner's guide.* Washington, DC, World Bank.

[5] Wagstaff, A. 2007. *Social Health Insurance Reexamined.* Washington, World Bank Policy Research Working Paper 4111, http://www-wds.worldbank.org/external/default/WDSContent Server/IW3P/IB/2007/01/09/000016406_20070109161148/Rendered /PDF/wps4111.pdf [*Comparison of social insurance and taxation*]

[6] Ensor, T. 2008. *Transition to universal coverage in developing countries. Encyclopaedia of Public Health.* K.Heggenhougen (ed.) and G.Carrin (Economics & Finance ed.). New York, Elsevier.

[7] East African Community (EAC). 2014. *Situational analysis and Feasibility Study of Options for harmonisation of Social Health Protection systems towards Universal Health Coverage in the East*

African Community Partner States, Arusha: East African Community.

[8] Lu, C. et al. 2012. Towards Universal Health Coverage: An Evaluation of Rwanda Mutuelles in Its First Eight Years. *PLoS ONE* 7(6): e39282. doi:10.1371/journal.pone.0039282.

[9] Makaka, A., S. Breen & A. Binagwaho 2012. Universal health coverage in Rwanda: a report of innovations to increase enrolment in community-based health insurance. *Lancet:* DOI: http://dx.doi.org/10.1016/S0140-6736(13)60293-7.

[10] Rajkotia Y. 2007. *The political development of the Ghanaian National Health Insurance System: lessons in health governance.* Bethesda, MD: Health Systems 20/20 Project, Abt Associates Inc.

[11] Amporfu, E. 2013. Equity of the premium of the Ghanaian national health insurance scheme and the implication for achieving universal coverage. *International Journal for Equity in Health* (online). 12(4), (Accessed 10th November 2017), pp.1-9. Available from: http://www.equityhealthj.com/content/12/1/4.

[12] Mensah, S. A. 2012. The National Insurance Scheme in Ghana: Achievements and Challenges. In: Value for Money, Sustainability and Accountability in Health Sector. *A Conference of African Ministers of Finance and Health. 4th - 5th July 2012.* Tunis. Unpublished.

[13] *Organization of African Unity Abuja declaration on HIV/AIDS, tuberculosis, and other related infectious diseases (OAU/SPS/ABUJA/3).* http://www.un.org/ga/aids/pdf/abuja_declaration. pdf.

[14] Ministry of Health-Uganda. 2018. *Uganda Health Accounts: National Health Expenditure 2013/2014. Kampala*: MOH.

[15] Ministry of Health-Uganda 2015. *Health Sector Development Plan 2015/16 - 2019/20.* Kampala: MOH.

[16] Zikusooka, C. M., R. Kyomuhangi. 2008. *Private medical pre-payment and insurance schemes in Uganda: What can the proposed SHI policy learn from them?.* Equinet Discussion Paper 53.

[17] Uganda Legal Information Institute. 2017. *Insurance Amendment – Act 2011.* https://ulii.org/ug/legislation/act/2015/13-2 (Accessed on 16 Jan 2018).

[18] Derriennic, Y., R. P. Wolf and Kiwanuka-Mukiibi. 2005. *An assessment of Community Based Health Financing Activities in Uganda*. Bethesda, MD: The Partners for Health Reform *plus* Project, Abt Associates Inc.

[19] UCBHFA. 2014. *Strategic Plan 2013/2014 -2017/2018*. Kampala, Uganda.

[20] Carrin, G. 2003 *Community based Health Insurance Schemes in Developing Countries: facts, problems and perspectives,* Discussion Paper. Geneva, WHO.

[21] Lukwago, D. 2010. *Health spending in Uganda: Implication on the National minimum health care package*. Unpublished.

[22] Basaza, K. R., B. Criel and V. Van der Stuyft 2007. Low enrolment in Ugandan Community Health Insurance Schemes: Underlying causes and policy implications. *BMC Health Services Research,* 7:105.

[23] Ministry of Health, Uganda. 2019. *The National Health Insurance Bill.* Kampala, Uganda.

[24] The World Bank. 2016. *The Uganda Poverty Assessment Report*. New York; The World Bank Group.

[25] IRA, 2015. *Personal Communication from Insurance Regulatory Authority of Uganda.*

[26] Mwesigye, F., and M. Pearson. 1997. Kisiizi hospital health society: pioneering rural social health insurance. *Uganda Health Bulletin, Ministry of Health Journal,* 1(4), 60-64.

[27] Masiko, A. 1998. *Community-Based Health Financing - The Kisiizi experience can it be sustained?* A dissertation submitted for the award of Masters of Arts degree of Leeds University.

[28] Insurance Regulatory Authority of Uganda. 2017. *Annual Insurance Market Report 2016*. Kampala, IRA.

[29] Uganda Insurers Association. 2015. *2014 Annual Report*. Kampala, UIA.

[30] Uganda Insurers Association. 2016. *2015 Annual Report*. Kampala, UIA.

[31] Insurance Regulatory Authority of Uganda. *2017. Website.* www.ira.go.ug. (Accessed on 15th December 2017).

[32] Insurance Regulatory Authority. 2014. *Annual Insurance Market Report.* Kampala, IRA.

[33] Uganda Bureau of Statistics. 2016. *The National Population and Housing Census 2014 – Main Report*, Kampala, Uganda.

[34] Basaza, R., T. S. O'Connell., and I. Chapčáková,. 2013. Players and processes behind the national health insurance scheme: a case study of Uganda. *BMC Health Services Research;* 13:357. Accessed on line on 20th December 2017 from: http://www.biomedcentral.com/1472-6963/13/357.

[35] Goddard, M. 2015. *Competition in Healthcare: Good, Bad or Ugly?* Int J Health Policy Management; 4(9): 567–569.

[36] Pacific Prime. 2017. *Website.* Accessed on 20th December 2017 from https://www.pacificprime.com/country/africa/uganda-health-insurance/ .

[37] Among, B. 2009. *Microcare in financial crisis.* New Vision, Uganda. www.newvision.co.ug (Accessed on 20th November 2017).

[38] Microcare- Uganda. 2010. *Financing Health through Communities.* http://www.un.org/esa/sustdev/publications/africa_casestudies/micro care.

[39] Zikusooka, C., Kwesiga, Lagony, 2014. Universal Health Coverage Assessment. *Global Network for Health Equity (GNHE).* http://funsalud.org.mx/gnhe/Contact.html.

[40] A-etna. 2017. *Website*: Accessed on 20th December 2017 from https://www.aetnainternational.com/en/about-us/explore/living-abroad/culture-lifestyle/health-care-quality-in-africa.html.

[41] Daily Monitor. 2016. *Insurance industry to grow by 8.2% - report.* Accessed on 20th December 2017: http://www.monitor.co.ug/Business/Insurance-industry-grow-8-2--report. IAA. 2017. *Website.* Accessed on 21st December 2017 from: http://iaa.img.co.ug/hsps/.

[42] IAA. 2017. *Website.* Accessed on 21st December 2017 from: http://iaa.img.co.ug/hsps/

[43] Ministry of Finance, Planning and Economic Development. 2015. *Continuous stock-outs of medical supplies in Uganda: What are the root causes?* BMAU Briefing Paper (15/15). Kampala, MFPED.

[44] Jubilee Insurance. 2018. *Website*: https://jubileeinsurance.com/ug/ (Accessed on 25th June 2018).

In: The Journey …
Editors: Robert Basaza et al.
ISBN: 978-1-53618-323-8

Chapter 7

HEALTHCARE FINANCING REFORMS IN GHANA: KEY LESSONS FOR UNIVERSAL HEALTH INSURANCE COVERAGE IN UGANDA

***Samuel G. Anarwat*[1,*] *and Donald S. Shepard*[2]**
[1]University for Development Studies, Tamale, Ghana
[2]Brandeis University, MA, US

ABSTRACT

Background

Universal health insurance coverage has been proven to reduce catastrophic episodes of health care at the point of delivery to millions of households. Following the health care delivery and access challenge, Ghana established its National Health Insurance Scheme (NHIS) in 2003 with the passing of the National Health Insurance bill into law (Act 650, 2003). The main goal of the NHIS was a pro-poor health financing policy

* Corresponding Author's E-mail: anarwat@gmail.com.

intervention to provide health care to all residents of the country. Since its establishment, the NHIS has achieved a steady growth of up to 41% population coverage in 2016, but with equity and financial sustainability challenges. We present detailed pathways of the health financing reform and universal health insurance in Ghana.

Purpose

This chapter presents the detailed experience of Ghana's health care financing pathways, the challenges, the best practices and lessons learned for possible replication in the establishment of Universal Health Insurance in Uganda and other similar settings.

Methods

This paper used mixed methods approach. We conducted an extensive desk review of relevant literature about Ghana's NHIS, 12 in-depth interviews with selected healthcare providers, 20 in-depth interviews and focus group discussions with key personnel and management of the National Health Insurance Authority, Ministry of Health, and Ghana Health Services.

Findings

The study revealed very useful lessons in political economy of health financing in Ghana, the implementation processes, and governance, equity and sustainability challenges of the NHIS. Appropriate legislation, social solidarity, strong political will, tax funding and safety net for the poor and vulnerable are necessary determinants of a successful NHIS. Adopting appropriate principles such as solidarity, cross-subsidization, equity and empowerment of insured members to have a voice in the scheme and avoiding excessive domestic politicization of a health insurance scheme can effectively enhance its success. The study also found that adopting fee-for-service payment method without effective control measures can be a recipe for healthcare provider fraud. However, the capitation payment method engenders shared responsibilities between the provider, the purchaser and the patients, hence a triple win, when implemented with effective monitoring mechanisms. Finally, while the study found generous health insurance benefits package, and premium exemptions for the vulnerable as cardinal principles of a pro-poor health insurance scheme, the paradox is that these same measures, if not effectively managed, can increase the costs of the NHIS and cause its collapse.

Conclusion

The Ghana's NHIS model shows that countries do not need huge resources or a gold standard plan before establishing a universal health insurance scheme. With a combination of appropriate legislation, and tax funding mechanism coupled with strong political will, a national health insurance scheme can be established using the learning by doing approach while adopting corrective measures on its path to success. This Ghana NHIS model is a practical example for replication in other developing, and even advanced countries. These lessons learned from Ghana's NHIS could serve as guiding principles for Uganda and the rest of the East African Community in their quest for universal health insurance schemes.

ABBREVIATIONS

CBHIS	Community–Based Health Insurance Scheme;
CHAG	Christian Health Association of Ghana;
CHPS	Community Health Planning and Services;
DANIDA	Danish International Development Agency;
DFID	Department for International Development;
ERP	Economic Recovery Programme;
FGD	Focus Group Discussion;
GDP	Gross Domestic Product (National Income);
G-DRG	Ghana Diagnostic Related Group;
GHS	Ghana Health Service;
GSS	Ghana Statistical Service;
IMF	International Monetary Fund;
LI	Legislative Instrument;
MHO	Mutual Health Organization;
MOH	Ministry of Health;
NDC	National Democratic Congress;
NHIA	National Health Insurance Authority;

NHIC	National Health Insurance Council;
NHIS	National Health Insurance Scheme;
NHS	National Health Service;
NPP	New Patriotic Party;
OOP	Out-of-Pocket Payment;
SAP	Structural Adjustment Program;
SDG	Sustainable Development Goals;
SES	Socio-Economic Status;
UHC	Universal Health Coverage;
UN	United Nations;
USAID	United States Agency for International Development;
VAT	Value Added Tax;
WHO	World Health Organization.

INTRODUCTION

Universal health insurance coverage has been proven to reduce catastrophic episodes of health care at the point of delivery to millions of households (WHO, 2010). Following the health care delivery and access challenges Ghana established its National Health Insurance Scheme (NHIS) in 2003 with the passing of the National Health Insurance bill into law (Act 650, 2003). The main goal of the NHIS was a pro-poor health financing policy intervention to provide health care to all residents of the country (MOH, 2004). Since its establishment, the NHIS has achieved a steady growth of up to 41% population coverage in 2016 but with equity and financial sustainability challenges. Nonetheless, Ghana's NHIS model is one good practice example for replication in other developing, and even advanced countries (NHIA, 2016).

This chapter presents an exposé of the key health care financing policies and strategies that have been adopted by various governments of Ghana to improve quality healthcare access to its residents. The chapter paints a picture of Ghana's situation, in health, politically and economically. It later details the National Health Insurance Scheme and the lessons that might be useful for a country like Uganda. As a learning strategy, the chapter concludes and provides recommendations for Uganda for adaptation of the best practices based on Ghana's NHIS model, and to tread cautiously on her own path towards implementation and sustainability of Uganda's NHIS, using the red and green flags of Ghana's NHIS as a guide.

The History and Political Economy of Ghana

Ghana experimented and adopted various health care financing policies in an attempt to provide health care for its residents. These policies which spanned free healthcare, cost sharing, user fees, community based-health insurance and the current social health insurance scheme, all had their strengths and challenges.

Before Ghana's political independence of 1957, the health care financing policies were modeled along the lines of social policy and equity theories with the aim of providing financial and geographic access to quality health care service. Various political administrations in Ghana adopted varied health care financing policies to provide equitable and affordable health care for residents. The initial policy that was implemented was the National Health Services (NHS) system, which provided free health care for all Ghanaian residents. This policy was made possible, probably, because Ghana had favorable population dynamics and a very good economic gradient.

In the late 1950s through the 1960s, Ghana experienced 100% public financed healthcare delivery with no direct out-of-pocket payment for health services. This free public health care financed policy was also made possible because development resources were commensurate with the population of Ghana at the time. This free healthcare policy was implemented in tandem with the first seven-year national development plan (1963-1970) which emphasized a massive expansion of health infrastructure and services to various communities across the country. The financial access to health care goal was met as residents did not have to pay at the point of service, but geographical access remained a problem. Most of the health personnel remained in the urban sectors while the rural areas remained without health personnel (Yeboah, 2003).

In the 1970s, however, when the population started growing amidst dwindling national resources, the free health service policy could not be sustained. In the midst of major political transitions, the country experienced economic stagnation, and the tax-based financed NHS could not be supported. Different military and civilian governments based on a trial- and-error system, adopted alternative policies from across peculiar countries in the Far East to revamp the health financing policy. Consequently, the government experimented minimal user-fees in 1971 to finance healthcare as a way of cost recovery for hospital procedures and overheads. This policy was supported and implemented under the Hospital Fees Decree of 1969 which was later amended in 1971 as the Hospital Fees Act, 1971 (Owusu-Sekyere & Bagah, 2014).

The health delivery and financing situation worsened in the early 1980s when the country experienced severe economic crisis. In the quest for a better alternative health policy to salvage the deplorable health situation and improve the health status of the nation, the then government adopted the Structural Adjustment Program (SAP) also known as Economic Recovery Program (ERP) imposed on developing countries by the Bretton Woods institutions namely; the International Monetary Fund (IMF) and the World Bank in the late 1970s and early 1980s with all the harsh conditionalities. The government had to adopt ERP to salvage the country of the negative economic growth. The situation in the health sector during that period was characterized by poor health services and most health facilities did not have essential health services such as medicine, consumables, and surgical materials. In public health services, there was a shortage of human resources for health as a result of the brain drain of professional health workers such as doctors and nurses to Europe and America (Agyepong & Adjei, 2008).

The adoption of the World Bank's ERP and later the SAP in 1983 had a severe turning effect on most sectors of the economy, especially, the agriculture and health sectors leading to a sharp decline in productivity, export revenues, high inflationary pressures and increased unemployment as many workers had to be retrenched and many public facilities including health units had to be privatized (Asenso -Okyere, Osei Akoto, Anum, & Appiah, 1997). The central argument put forward by the IMF for this policy was to help the government inject economic sanity into the economy through effective pricing, withdrawals of subsidies, domestic and external trade liberalization. Scholars further recount that the SAP introduced various aspects of deregulation into the economy, proposed reducing the size of the state in favor of the private sector, which led to retrenchment of many public-sector workers and drastic budget cuts in social services including government expenditure on healthcare which largely affected health service delivery and access in the country (Owusu-Sekyere & Bagah, 2014).

User Fees ("Cash and Carry") Health Financing Policy

Following the economic downturn and the worsening situation in the healthcare sector in the country, the government was compelled to adopt the hospital user-fees as a health care financing policy from 1980 to 1985. The user fees syndrome reached its peak in 1985 when, as a result of the IMF and World Bank's unpopular "cash and carry system" patients had to pay for services at the point of delivery. Without cash, "no service would be delivered even including accident and emergency cases. The system was introduced "en masse" in all public health facilities" (Agyepong & Adjei, 2008). The "Cash and Carry" policy had positive intended consequences of cost recovery at the public health facilities as a result of the worsening economic crises.

Evidence shows that the policy was associated with increased financial resource mobilization and infrastructural development at many public health facilities. There was a disconnect between policy and practice. Patients' accounts revealed that the policy resulted in devastating unintended consequences: many patients were detained in hospital for inability to pay their bills and many lost their lives because they were denied services (Nyonator & Kutzin, 1999; Waddington & Enyimayew, 1989).The user fees policy for all medical conditions except specified communicable diseases, plunged the nation into another catastrophic health situation which registered countless deaths, especially among the poor in Ghana (Government of Ghana Ministry of Health, 2014).

The World Bank's arguments for the introduction of user fees had been that the policy would generate revenue, promote efficiency, foster equity and enhance sustainability (Nyman, 1999). Another school of thought that user-fees would further impoverish the poor and deny them access to health care, as they would not be able to afford it at the point of care, seemed to be visible at that time. To justify this argument and to mitigate the effects of the policy on the poor, the user fees exemptions policy was introduced in public hospitals in which all children under-five, the aged and certain communicable disease like tuberculosis were exempted from fee payment. Later, pregnant women were also exempted from the user-fee- payment.

Evidence indicates that the guidelines and the package of the exemption policy were not clearly specified and paved way for wide spread corruption and discretionary measures in the implementation of the policy. It also suffered from inadequate funding, managerial and operational challenges which together led to the inefficiencies and limited success. As a result, this policy failed to eliminate the financial barriers to healthcare access (Government of Ghana, Ministry of Health, 2007).

Despite technological advancement in health and numerous public health interventions and health promotion, the Ministry of Health (Ghana) reports that not only were communicable diseases the leading cause of morbidity and mortality from the early 2000s to 2008 but also posed major financial and emotional burdens on households. Even though access to medication (drugs) and consumables were improving in both public and private health facilities, there were cost inefficiencies as a result of high drug prices. A worrying phenomenon was the quality of medications in the pharmaceutical industry as fake medications were increasingly flooding the market. The Food and Drug Board was finding a hard time to curb this problem due to the numerous roots and strategies the drug syndicate were using to get those fake medications into the country. The quality of healthcare and health worker attitudes remained a challenge to health care. The quality of care, workers' performance, and productivity were below standard. There were poor attitudes toward patients resulting in low patient access mostly in rural areas, and among the poor, especially in the Northern regions (Saleh, 2013).The good news, however, was that most of the top killer diseases in Ghana are preventable. Implementing sound policies and leveraging available financial and human capital toward health care promotion and prevention would yield much dividends in the health care provision in Ghana (Anarwat, 2012).

Ghana's Current Healthcare System

The Ghana health system is composed of the Ministry of Health as the policy-making body with the Ghana Health Service as a sub-ordinate body and the executing agency of the Ghana health policy. Other agencies under the MOH are the National Health Insurance Authority in charge of the NHIS.

The key actors in the health financing reforms were teaching hospitals which administer tertiary care, Ghana Medical and Dental Council, Pharmaceutical Council, Ghana Registered Nurses, and Midwives Council, and the Christian Health Association of Ghana (CHAG), in charge of not-for -profit Christian hospitals (doctors and nurses paid by government). Other agencies under the MOH include the Traditional Medicine Association (also gaining grounds and has a sector office under the MOH) and the private hospitals. The Ministry of Health has oversight responsibilities over all these agencies. The main role of the Ministry of Health is policy and regulation (Republic of Ghana, Ministry of Health, 2015). Health services are decentralized to the 170 districts in Ghana, and each district has a District Health Directorate headed by a District Director of Health Service. At the remote communities, there are the Community Health Planning and Service (CHPS) compounds where community health nurses live with the people in selected communities and take care of the health needs of the community, at least, for basic health services, while referring serious cases to the district or regional hospitals depending on the condition of the patient.

Health service delivery is designed to operate through the gate-keeper system. This means that the first point of call for health service is CHPS compound or the community health center, then referral to the district hospital through to the regional hospital and finally to the teaching hospitals. This is how the gatekeeper system is supposed to function but, in reality, it is not the case; patients have a choice of providers and can, therefore, select any provider at any facility level. It is hoped that, with the introduction of the capitation payment method and the preferred primary care providers system, the gatekeeper system may work, to reduce pressures on the specialized hospitals for simple ailments that can be easily treated at the CHPS compounds and community health centres.

METHODOLOGY

This paper used mixed methods approach. The authors conducted extensive desk review of relevant literature on Ghana's NHIS, focus group discussions (FGD), in-depth interviews with 12 selected health providers, 20 key personnel and management of the National Health Insurance Authority, Ministry of Health, and Ghana Health Services.

FINDINGS AND DISCUSSION

Exposé of Health Insurance in Ghana: Pathways and Challenges

The idea of introducing health insurance in Ghana as an alternative health care financing was conceived out of the challenges of the health care system of the time: the near collapse of the health care system and the inhumane out-of-pocket health care financing at the point of delivery dubbed "Cash and Carry" (Atim & Sock, 2000).

Community-Based Health Insurance Schemes in Ghana

Health insurance in Ghana started as community-based health insurance, termed as Mutual Health Organizations (MHOs). This idea of community-based health insurance was borne out of compassion to finance health care for the dying patients in rural communities. This idea of health insurance to finance patients, especially in-patients, was a novelty of the Catholic Diocese of the Sunyani District. The Catholic Diocese piloted a health facility-based in-patient district health insurance scheme in the Nkoranza District (Brong Ahafo Region-Ghana) by the Saint Theresa's Mission Hospital in Nkoranza in 1992 (Atim & Sock, 2000). The Nkoranza community district health insurance scheme was established out of compassion to help the rural poor (mostly farmers) in the district who could not afford to pay for health care at the point of delivery. From a humble beginning, using solidarity, a social value of the community, the Nkoranza scheme covered a third of the population of the district in a spate of less than ten years from 1992 to 2000 (Atim & Sock, 2000). The enormous successes and the testimonies of patients and their families inspired stakeholders in health care such as the MOH, Ghana Health Services (GHS) to think of health insurance as a viable alternative for health care financing. The Nkoranza Health Insurance Scheme, though had many challenges in its implementation, provided the needed evidence and impetus, which paved the way for the exploration and establishment of community-based health financing schemes in various kinds and magnitude in Ghana. Development partners, especially, DANIDA, and USAID through their Partnerships for Health Reform Plus Project, played an instrumental role in the promotion of community-based, faith-based, and employer-based health insurance schemes dotted all over Ghana, especially, the BrongAhafo, Northern, Upper West, Eastern and Greater Accra regions (Atim, Grey, Apoya, Anie, & Aikins, 2001)

Background of Ghana's National Health Insurance Scheme

The NHIS was established in 2003 following the passing of an Act of parliament (Act 650, 2003) to enable the implementation of a comprehensive, universal and pro-poor health insurance scheme for all residents of Ghana as a better alternative to abolishing out-of-pocket health care financing policy (Republic of Ghana, 2010). The establishment of the NHIS was necessitated by the health care financing policy at the time as discussed under "user fees –health financing policy" (Nyonator & Kutzin, 1999; Waddington & Enyimayew, 1989).

There was ample evidence from the experience of the pilot implementation of health insurance schemes and Community-based Health Insurance Schemes (CBHIS) and HMOs in Ghana (Atim et al, 2001; Blanchet and Acheampong, 2013) as well as international best practices of health insurance, especially from WHO which showed that health insurance could serve as a better alternative to provide financial protection to the populations. Almost all major political parties in Ghana had made it their campaign promise (as was detailed in their manifestos) to establish the NHIS and abolish the out-of-pocket (OOP) –User –fee payment method (Agyepong and Adjei, 2008).

The governing National Democratic Congress (NDC) lost the election to the leading opposition party, National Patriotic Party (NPP) in the 2000 elections. The foundations for National Health Insurance had already been laid but the giant step to move forward with a single unified payer NHIS was lacking. There was pressure from the masses for NPP to deliver its campaign promise of establishing the NHIS. Even though the foundation for health Insurance had been laid through the experience of CBHIS in Ghana, there were no actuarial studies to determine premiums and feasibility of the NHIS. Additionaly, was no immediate funding for the establishment of the NHIS. The scheme was to be funded by informal sector members' premium of GHS 7.2, 2.5% national health insurance levy and to be collected as value added tax on goods and services, including2.5% formal sector workers' social security and national health insurance trust contribution. This money was to be taken directly from the formal sector workers' pension fund (Agyepong & Adjei, 2008).

A committee of experts from the Ministry of Health including a traditional health practitioner was established to oversee the drafting of the NHIS bill. The bill was sent to parliament and hurriedly passed into law in 2003 before the 2004 election. The NHIS was established but the question then was how to finance it going forward (Agyepong & Adjei, 2008).

Legal Framework

The National Health Insurance Scheme (NHIS) is governed by two major Acts of Parliament: the initial Act 650, 2003 and the revised Act 852, 2012 with its accompanying legislative instruments that guide the implementation processes. The initial NHIS law, Act 650, 2003, set up the legal and institutional framework for the establishment of the semi-autonomous district mutual health insurance schemes with an independent board of directors and community committees of the Mutual Health Insurance Schemes. It also established the private voluntary and private commercial schemes operating in parallel. A key feature of NHIS Act 650, 2003 was that it exempted children under 18 years of age from paying premium subject to at least one parent being a member of the scheme. Each district mutual health insurance scheme operated independently with oversight responsibilities from the National Health Insurance Council. Act 852, 2012 consolidated all the over 145 disjointed district mutual health insurance schemes and the voluntary mutual health organizations into a single unified payer NHIS. It also established the National Health Insurance Authority (NHIA), a subsidiary of the Ministry of Health to govern the nationwide unified NHIS with ten regional offices and over 140 district offices. One of the key features of NHIS Act 852, 2012 is that it decoupled children (up to 17 years) from their parents and exempted them from paying a premium, which meant that the condition that required at least one of the parents to be a member of the NHIS was no longer necessary. In addition, it consolidated all the schemes under one single payer NHIS with one governance and administrative system and the power to accredit health care providers (Republic of Ghana, NHIS Act 852, 2012).

Governance

Governance of the NHIS is operationalized in this study as the institutional and administrative arrangements, functions, responsibilities, and the existing interconnections between the NHIA and its strategic partners and stakeholders. It also includes systems, and routine operations of the NHIA, the checks and balances, the relationships among various directorates, the regional and operational offices at the district level and the various mechanisms put in place to ensure accountability, stewardship and strategic direction of the NHIS.

The findings of the study indicate that the NHIA is the regulator of the NHIS. The NHIA has established systems based on the governing laws including administrative procedures, registration and enrollment process of members, provider payment methods, reporting, financial and internal management systems.

Good governance of the NHIA is key to achieving efficiency, quality health care to members of the scheme, equity in coverage and financial risk protection, cost containment and sustainability of the scheme. The evidence gathered showed that, the NHIA has a functioning administrative structure with a world-class head office complex. However, it has 17 different directorates including claims, financing, administration and human resource, provider payment, enrollment and regional operations. Other directorates are policy research, monitoring and evaluation, management information systems, clinical audit, corporate affairs, actuarial directorate, among others. Besides, there are 10 regional offices and over 130 district offices across the length and breadth of the country. In as much as these different directorates may be necessary, there is less coordination and information sharing among them which probably leads to duplication of efforts and resources (NHIA, 2016).

The NHIA had over 3,000 employees who superintend over the operations of the NHIS, making it one of the largest employers in Ghana (NHIA, 2016). Nonetheless, the findings suggest that the number of employees and technical experts are not enough to embark on efficient operations, monitoring and claims management of the scheme. The findings show that governance of the NHIS could be rated as good which has led to the remarkable success of the scheme. However, persistent politicization of the scheme and a few administrative lapses which are forestalling its growth and purchasing functions, need improvement (Anarwat, 2018).

Domestic Political Considerations

The study revealed that domestic political issues have influenced the scheme both positively and negatively. For instance, the results showed a strong political will and government support to strengthen the scheme. Many opposition parties expressed concerns in various forms regarding their firm support for the growth and sustainability of the NHIS if they were given the nod to rule. The government has on critical times bailed-out the NHIS through financial injection to forestall its collapse, given the important role it plays in health care financing. The study found the strong political will and government support a strong pillar for the growth and success of the NHIS, which other developing countries can emulate to improve their health insurance schemes.

The results also suggest that domestic political influence has significantly affected the NHIS negatively in terms of enrollment and public confidence in the scheme. However, findings from both the focus group discussions (FGDs) and policy interviews showed that, though the NHIS enjoys strong political will and most governments and opposition parties heralded it as a flagship social intervention project which could promote universal health coverage in Ghana, unintended consequences overshadowed the positive political will. For instance, the results revealed frequent changes of staff and management of the scheme whenever there was a political regime change which invariably disrupted the continuity and smooth running of the scheme due to inexperience and loss of internal organizational memories. One of the FGD participants expressed that:

> "I think that politics play a negative effect on NHIS because when a new government is elected they change most of the NHIS officials who were initially there and bring their own party members and this is affecting the progress of the scheme. Many technical experts of the NHIS have been relieved of their post due to change of political regimes, and new personnel brought in to start afresh. All these affect the smooth running of the NHIS" (FGD of staff of NHIS).

An account was provided that there have been five changes of the Chief Executive Officers (CEOs) of the NHIS since its inception in 2013, which has affected its strategy and vision and implicitly lowered the speedy growth of the scheme. These changes have not only come with administrative challenges but also financial and cost implications. A recent (2017) personal communication with key management staff of the NHIS revealed that over 200 personnel of the NHIS perceived to be loyal to the previous regime have been relieved of their various posts to be replaced by new personnel loyal to the current regime. This kind of organizational behavior affects the smooth operations of the scheme, creates tension among the staff and also retards its progress.

Sources of Funding

The NHIS is mainly financed through the Value Added Tax on goods and services (74%). There is a mandatory health insurance levy of 2.5% deduction from formal sector workers' social security contribution (20%) and 3% from health insurance premiums. The premium charged which ranges from GHS 7.20 (3%) equivalent of only UDS 4.00 minimum and GHS 48.00 equivalent of GHS 25.00 per annum in 2003, was based on socio-economic status (Republic of Ghana, 2010). Other relevant sources of funding are investment and contributions from donors (NHIS Act 650, NHIS

Act 852). However, due to lack of reliable data and the cumbersome nature of identifying the poor, almost all schemes charge a flat rate of Ghc7.20 and many poor are not exempted (Jehu-Appiah, Aryeetey, Spaan, & Agyepong, 2010). The NHIS comprises 145 district mutual health insurance schemes out of the 216 districts in Ghana.

Benefits Package

The Ministry of Health report, 2004, NHIS Act 650, 2003, Act 852, 2012, and National Health Insurance Scheme report, 2015 reveal that NHIS covers about 95% of all the common health cases in Ghana. These include, in broader terms:

Out-Patient (OP) Services

These are consultations and reviews: requested investigations including laboratory, x-rays, and ultra-sounds; medication, primarily prescription medications on the NHIS essential medicines list; treatment of HIV/AIDS symptomatic opportunistic infections; simple surgeries and physiotherapy.

In–Patient (IP) Services

These are general and specialty care, requested investigations including x-ray and ultra-sound, medication on the NHIS prescribed medication list, cervical breast cancer treatment, surgery, feeding, and admission accommodation in the general wards.

Maternity Care

Include antenatal, postnatal, normal and assisted deliveries and caesarian sections.

Eye Care Services, Emergency Care, and Oral Health Services

It is worthy stating that the availability of, and access to these services is dependent on the type of health facility visited but the gatekeeper system allows for referral to higher facilities, both public and private, to receive the needed care. However, the benefit package excludes HIV/AIDS antiretroviral therapy, hearing aids, dentures, and complicated surgeries, which implies that the poor are denied healthcare of this kind of problems because they may not be able to afford to pay out-of-pocket.

Provider Payment Methods

The NHIS pays providers for the health care services rendered through different payment methods namely, fee-for-service, Ghana diagnostic related groupings (G-DRG) and health care capitation. With the fee-for-service payment method, providers bill each itemized service provided from consultation, laboratory test, to medication at the pharmacy. This is the worse form of provider payment because all the responsibility of payment rests on the patient and the purchaser. Ghana's NHIS practiced the fee-for-service provider payment method at the initial stages of the NHIS. This resulted in huge claims costs to the NHIS due to health care provider fraud (NHIA, 2016). This method of payment, though flexible and easy, is a red flag that should be avoided in the national health insurance schemes for Uganda or similar settings.

The capitation payment method is the best method of health care provider payment because it promotes shared responsibilities among the provider, the patient and the purchaser, and all win (the triple-win of capitation) (Sheiber, Cashin, Saleh, & Lavado 2012). However, with this method, if strong control measures are not put in place to monitor health care providers, quality could be compromised. It is important to note that there is no perfect health care payment method. They all have their pros and cons. Therefore, the choice of the payment method should be contextual.

Guiding Design Principles

The NHIS was initially designed based on ten interrelated principles taking into consideration the political and social economy of the time (Government of Ghana, Ministry of Health, 2004). These principles were equity, risk-equalization, cross-subsidization, quality care, solidarity, efficiency in premium (members' contribution) collection and claims administration, community or member-ownership, partnership, re-insurance and sustainability. These principles were the very foundation of the NHIS. They are the gold standards of health financing schemes. These ten operational principles of health insurance have been approximated by a few industrialized countries, but these WHO standards have not all been realized in developing countries. Nevertheless, they serve as a guide towards improvement. For this study, the design principles are operationalized:

Equity

The equity principle under the NHIS means everybody registered under the scheme should have access to the minimum benefits package irrespective of the person's socio-economic background. It also means that everyone resident in Ghana can join the NHIS without discrimination and that health insurance should be at the doorstep of every resident in Ghana. It equally implies that health insurance should be available and affordable to members at all times in order not to deny members access to health care at the point of need. It also means both the poor and the rich, rural dwellers and urban residents should all have equal opportunity to register with the NHIS according to their abilities and should all have readily available access to essential health care services, irrespective of location and income levels, socio-economic and demographic status. In this study, equity is assessed both qualitatively and quantitatively.

Risk Equalization

Risk equalization means that the MOH and NHIS will ensure that the disease burden and patterns of mortality serve as one of the bases for allocating financial resources to geographical areas of the country as the cost of care varies depending on the disease burden of each area. Besides, the disease burden correlates positively with poverty; therefore, a risk equalization formula is developed to make up the cost difference based on the minimum contribution levels. This also means that both members with higher risk-burdens of disease, for instance, those insured members with chronic diseases would all be covered by the NHIS under the same terms and conditions as the healthy insured members. This is a nicely calved principle on paper but the reality is that no risk-equalization formula has been developed for the allocation of resources based on geographical areas and burden of disease. At best, we can say allocation of resources is based on population dynamics and emergencies. A key challenge is that regions with resources, especially the southern sector of Ghana and the urban centers have some capacities to generate internal income to complement government effort. However, regions in the northern part are very poor and have little capacity for internal resource generation (Republic of Ghana, Ministry of Health, 2015; Anarwat S. G., 2018).

Cross-Subsidization

The cross-subsidization principle implies contribution (premium) should be based on the ability to pay. Therefore, the rich pay more while the poor pay less. It also avoids adverse selection and ensures that those with a high risk of falling ill, the sick and the healthy, all contribute to the scheme. In other words, the rich cross-subsidize the poor and the vulnerable, the healthy cross-subsidize the sick, and the economically active cross-subsidize for children and the aged. The reality is that we can consider the situation of cross-subsidization as a "half-full bottle rather than a half-empty bottle. To some extent, there is cross-subsidization in terms of premium payments and the value-added tax financing of the NHIS. People in the poor regions pay a little less premium than people in the endowed region. Also, the poor, the pensioners, children under 18 years and pregnant women are all premium-exempt. Again, both the sick and the healthy enroll in the NHIS. However, the one month only waiting period for health benefits creates a loophole for the sick to enroll more because of their vulnerability, and paradoxically, the healthy think they are fit and do not need health insurance, hence more adverse selection and less cross-subsidization (Government of Ghana, Ministry of Health, 2016; Anarwat S. G., 2018).

Quality of Care

All things being equal, patients are more likely to use health care that they perceive to be of quality than one that is of less quality. The principle of quality care under the NHIS means value for money. Perceived quality of health care means increased propensity to use health care services, which also is linked to health care access while poor quality of care is a barrier to access. Hence, under this principle, NHIS will ensure that the health care providers will provide quality services within the prescribed benefits package. Quality is also time-variant, which means health care services should be provided to patients at the point of need in real time. The reality on the ground is that patients perceive the services provided under the NHIS as poor quality. Interviews with providers confirmed poor quality services, especially, in the rural areas because of less health facilities, medicines and personnel, and urban centers because of long waiting time, doctor absenteeism and "moonlighting as well as poor health workers' attitude towards patients. Some efforts are being put in place by the Ghana Health Service, such as quality controls and quality assurance surveys, and disciplinary actions against unprofessional acts of personnel. The NHIA accredits health facilities and carries out monitoring and evaluation visits to ensure quality and compliance to guidelines, and in some cases, sanctions some non-performing health facilities. However, there is much room for improvement in quality health delivery in Ghana (Government of Ghana, Minsitry of Health, 2016).

Solidarity

Solidarity is a desired virtue in Social Health Insurance. Health insurance thrives on the principle of everybody being his "neighbors' keeper" as the health status of an individual is inter-linked, especially, when dealing with communicable diseases which are the main causes of morbidity in Ghana. The solidarity principle means that community members are helping one another by fighting diseases and supporting one another collectively to have access to quality health care: the rich supporting the poor and the strong supporting the vulnerable besides all registering in the NHIS without anyone left out.

The idea of health insurance in Ghana dates back to the early 1980s and the early 1990s. Though, national health insurance is seemingly new, the concept of social insurance could be traced back to the cultural values and practices of the people of Ghana through their communal self-help practices. The community members practiced strong solidarity measures by mobilizing material and human resources to help each other in times of sickness, bereavement, child delivery and naming ceremonies, and communal farming dubbed Nnoboa" in the local Akan language and "Kpaguur" in the local Bimoba language. This solidarity measure and self-help cultural practice was common in almost all cultures in Ghana. It could, therefore, be said that the concept of health insurance was part of the cultural values of the people of Ghana. These already existing cultural practices of self-help might have facilitated the easy introduction and formation of MHOs in Ghana, a precursor to the NHIS (Anarwat S. G., 2018).

Efficiency in the Collection of Contributions and Claims Administration

This principle ensures that the NHIS adopts a pragmatic system of premium collection and claims administration to build a sustainable fund for the scheme as well as effective and efficient reimbursement of providers for services rendered. The efficiency principle looks at both the supply and the demand or purchasing sides. This also means there should be an efficient use of health insurance funds: cost containment measures put in place in the management of health insurance funds, reduction in internal fraud and misappropriation of funds within the NHIS; and external fraud and moral hazards from providers to ensure efficiency gains. Inefficiencies have been the bane of the NHIS and a major cost driver. There have been instances of corruption in the management of NHIS funds, provider fraud and moral hazards as revealed by the interview with health providers and the management of the NHIA. Measures have been put in place to sanction perpetrators of NHIS fraud and suspend perpetrators of health care provider fraud under the NHIS (Government of Ghana, Minsitry of Health, 2016).

Community or Member Ownership

This principle is vital to ensure participation and enrollment into the NHIS. Under the scheme, members of the NHIS are part owners of the scheme and therefore, have a common voice in the management. Not only are they part owners and have a voice, but they also establish channels where members' grievances can be aired and addressed. Community ownership promotes participation thereby bringing in members' perspective of quality of care in the delivery process and demand accountability. Evidence from focus group discussions with beneficiaries suggest that members do not consider themselves as part owners of the NHIS because they have no voice in the running of the NHIS. The NHIS contracted a third-party call center in the capital city of Accra but it was not very efficient as they only received complaints but had no power to address members' concerns. There is a proposition to establish patient protection and conflict resolution centers in at least each of the 10 regions in Ghana (Anarwat S. G., 2018).

Partnership

The partnership principle means the government is a strategic partner to the scheme for the sustainability. The scheme being a pro-poor policy, government is required to provide central funds to bridge the gap that may result from the expected contribution level and the actual contributions. The government should provide safety-nets in the form of exemptions for the poor and the vulnerable under the NHIS such as payment of contribution on behalf the poor, the children under 18 years and the aged. Indeed, there are safety-nets in terms of premium exemptions for the poor and the government is a strategic purchaser through the NHIA and a strategic health care provider through the GHS.

Reinsurance

The principle of reinsurance implies that the government allocates central funds aside to recapitalize schemes in the event that the Mutual

Health Insurance Schemes run into the risk of bankruptcy owing to epidemics and other external shocks such as floods, civil wars and where claims (utilization costs) unexpectedly exceed revenues of the scheme. In recent times the government bailed the NHIS to pay some of its debts to health care providers to keep the NHIS running.

Sustainability

The sustainability principle explains how well the NHIS would be governed and managed, especially, in risk management and cost containment. This principle, therefore, ensures that the NHIA develops the human resource capacity, systems, and policies to ensure the financial sustainability of the NHIS (Ministry of Health, Ghana, 2004). A breach of any one or more of these principles create a leeway for the gradual breakdown of the system and the eventual collapse of the scheme if corrective monitoring mechanisms are not put in place. The study assesses the effective application, or otherwise, of these principles in the operations of the NHIS. After a decade and a half of successful implementation of the NHIS, the growth of the scheme coupled with increased utilization are far above revenue mobilization. In addition to corruption, health care provider fraud and management lapses have created a threatening financial sustainability challenge. Strategic measures such as increasing the premium, the NHIS levy and downward revision of the benefit package to give priority to primary health care and increasing "sin taxes" have been implemented to generate more revenue for the sustenance of the NHIS (Government of Ghana, Ministry of Health, 2016).

KEY LESSONS FROM GHANA FOR UHC IN UGANDA

Target 3.8 of the United Nations' Sustainable Development Goals (SDGs) seeks to promote universal access to health care: "Achieve universal health coverage, including financial risk protection, access to quality essential health care services and access to safe, quality and affordable essential medicines and vaccines for all." Related to the demand side factors of promoting access are the supply side variables of health infrastructure, training and retention of the health workforce, which are essential determinants of quality health care delivery in developing countries, including Uganda. Consequently, the SDG goal 3c aims at promoting strategic health financing training and capacity building and retention of the health workforce, an essential component of universal health coverage (United Nations General Assembly, 2015). These SDGs health goal and targets, though excellent on paper, are only necessary but not sufficient conditions to promote the needed health financing and universal health coverage in developing countries unless health policy actors and implementers, as well as health consumers, adopt pragmatic strategies to implement it. In effect, if Uganda is to achieve the set goals and targets of the SDGs by 2030, then strong health care financing and delivery policies need to be implemented. These policies may also include, but not limited to progressive tax financing and other fund pooling for the establishment of its national health insurance scheme. Uganda could learn from its peer countries like Ghana and Rwanda which have vibrant and well-functioning national health insurance models. The political economy of health financing in Ghana, including best practices and lessons learned are adequately outlined in this chapter of the book for adaption and possible replication for the establishment and growth of the Ugandan National Health Insurance Scheme. In the next section the success factors of Ghana's NHIS are presented.

Success Factors of Ghana's NHIS for Adaptation

Ghana's NHIS has been internationally acclaimed as a "global best practice of social health insurance (Schieber, Cashin et al, 2012). Ghana's NHIS achieved moderate success since its establishment in 2003, recording a phenomenal 41% population coverage in 2016. Within the first five years of its implementation, the NHIS achieved an enrollment rate of more than two –thirds of the population and generated enough funds from multiple sources to finance the scheme, according to the NHIA (MOH, 2016). In this section we expound on the key factors behind the successes and the challenges in Ghana's NHIS to serve as valuable lessons for replication in Uganda, in particular, and East African Community as a whole, in their quest for social health insurance and universal health coverage.

History of Solidarity

The NHIS evolved from the few existing community-based health financing schemes which were spread around parts of the country. One of the major success factors of the NHIS was the existing solidarity practices in most cultures in Ghana. People saw each other as their brothers' keeper. This virtue of solidarity facilitated the formation of the community-based health financing schemes for health care, which were harmonized to form Ghana's NHIS. Since Ghana and Uganda have similar cultural values of solidarity, that could be a rallying point for the formation of community-based health insurance schemes, or a national health insurance scheme. There are various options opened to Uganda for the formation of the national health insurance scheme. 1) Promotion of voluntary community-based health insurance schemes which could later be harmonized to form a single-payer national health insurance scheme. 2) Employer-based social health insurance scheme which could be financed through employee and employer premium contribution at source which could serve as a rallying point for the formation of the national health insurance scheme. 3) An out-right legislation for the formation of a single national health insurance scheme to be financed partly through premiums and partly through taxes, 4) A mixture of voluntary community-based health insurance schemes and private commercial health insurance schemes with the government serving as a regulatory body of both. It is important to note that each of these types of health insurance schemes have their pros and cons, and, therefore, due diligence needs to be done to ascertain the viability and appropriateness before adopting any option.

Appropriate Legislation

Appropriate legislation needs to be promulgated to establish a national health insurance scheme. The legislation will spell-out the governance structure, the funding strategy, the precautionary and cost control measures, the functioning of the scheme, and the sustainability measures of the scheme. Ghana's NHIS was established through the successes of community-based health insurance schemes. The NHIS was made possible through a national health insurance legislation (National Health Insurance Act 650, 2003) which was enacted in 2003 to pave way for the establishment of a coordinated and comprehensive pro-poor social health insurance scheme. A legislative instrument (LI1809) was adopted in 2004 to guide the implementation of the scheme. The goal of the NHIS was to provide universal health insurance coverage for all people resident in Ghana by the 5th year of its establishment.

The NHIS law made provision for the establishment of three different types of health insurance schemes: district mutual health insurance scheme, private voluntary health insurance scheme and private commercial health insurance scheme. These three types of health insurance schemes form the national health insurance scheme. However, only the district mutual health insurance schemes are eligible for government subsidy of financing. In practice, the private voluntary mutual health insurance schemes (thus, the existing community based mutual health schemes) automatically merged to form the district mutual health insurance schemes-branches of the NHIS after the passing of the law. The private commercial health insurance schemes do need to apply for license from the National Health Insurance Council in order to set up and operate. Key lessons that Uganda and other peer countries should learn from the NHIS legislation is the manner in which it was passed. The NHIS legislation was rushed and passed amidst political turmoil. It was not given a full multi-partisan consideration before it was passed. The opposition party legislators staged a walk-out while the governing party passed the law by virtue of their simple majority in parliament. Many factors, including cost control measures and claims management measures among others were not taken into consideration before the bill was passed because it was rushed (Agyepong & Adjei, 2008).

Consequently, the legal framework of the scheme had several loopholes which militated against the smooth implementation and financial sustainability of the scheme. That notwithstanding, it is important to note that "half a loaf is better than none." The legislation had more positives than negatives. For example, the clause that allowed premium exemption for the aged, the vulnerable and children, and the clause that ensured the establishment of a national health insurance fund was phenomenal, and the government of the time needs commendation. If the Ugandan government is to pass any legislation for the establishment of a national health insurance scheme, it is imperative to ensure a multi-partisan approach and expert scrutiny of the bill before it is passed to ensure its effectiveness and appropriateness for smooth implementation and sustainability of the NHIS.

Governance

The NHIS is governed by a 15-member board which forms the National Health Insurance Council (NHIC). The NHIC manages the national health insurance fund, regulates the health insurance market and health services providers through licensing and accreditation. The NHIC is also responsible for providing subsidies to the district mutual health insurance scheme. The NHIA (Secretariat) is responsible for providing administrative support to the district mutual health insurance schemes and the NHIC. The secretariat has branch offices in all the 10 regions of Ghana.

Funding

The government explored multiple sources of funding to finance the NHIS such as 2.5% deduction from workers' social security contribution, 2.5% sales tax-Value Added Tax (VAT) for health insurance, GHS12.00 ($6.00) per annum, government budgetary allocation, donations and investment from accruals of the national health insurance fund. The population was already used to the value added tax payment system introduced to support tertiary education but the NHIS tax (levy) did not pass without public agitation.

Decentralized Local Government System

Another success point of the NHIS could be partly attributed to the existing well-organized functional decentralized local government systems and structure. It was very easy to implement the NHIS at the district level because of the already existing and function local government administrative systems including the district assemblies and the district health management teams, district hospitals and sub-district health centers and community clinics. A decentralized local government system could serve as a conduit which the Ugandan government could rely on to establish her NHIS.

The Role of CHAG/Mission Hospitals

The mission hospitals, organized under the umbrella of the Christian Health Association of Ghana (CHAG), played a significant role in the establishment and implementation of the community –based health insurance schemes which were later harmonized to form the single payer NHIS. The CHAG played a dual role by promoting the establishment of the community -based health insurance scheme in most of the districts where they operated, while the hospitals and health centers under the CHAG complemented government efforts by serving as health care providers of the NHIS. This is also a good lesson that could be adapted by the Ugandan government in the establishment and implementation of her NHIS because of the existing four religious medical bureaus: Catholic, Protestant, Muslim and Orthodox all of which have secretariats and run health centers and hospitals.

Learning by Doing Approach

One of the greatest characteristics that is promoting the growth the Ghana's NHIS is its *learning by doing approach* in its implementation. Ghana understood from the on-set that there cannot be a perfect system hence the adoption, of mostly experimental approach in its implementation, learning from the mistakes and adopting strategies to improve upon them. Consequently, there have been many pilot strategies, pilot studies, operational research, and feasibility studies using the results to improve upon the implementation of the scheme. Examples include: pilot capitation provider payment method, biometric registration and verification systems, instant printing of membership identification cards, manual and electronic claims systems, fee-for–service provider payment systems, and Ghana diagnostics related groupings (G-DRG) systems of payment. Some of these experiments and innovations can be adapted in the country-specific context of Uganda.

Strong Political Will

There was a strong political will towards the implementation of the NHIS. The government in power was determined to make NHIS succeed so as to retain power in the subsequent elections (NHIS was a campaign promise of the major political parties like the New Patriotic Party and the National Democratic Congress).

User-Fees Policy Challenges

The previous user-fee health policy was very "dehumanizing" as it was a financial access barrier to health care for residents, especially the poor in the informal sector. Hence, the introduction of the NHIS, where people prepaid insurance premium and received care without paying at the point of service was seen as a major health care relief for majority of families in Ghana.

Multifaceted Communication and Marketing Approach

Also, the government adopted multifaceted and all-involving marketing approaches such as social mobilization and marketing, community mobilization, local and national media campaigns, civil society, workers unions, NGOs, Ministry of Health's involvement at the national and grass-roots levels and also using renowned religious and traditional leaders to horn the NHIS message in their jurisdictions.

Development Partners

There was a strong donor support which facilitated the social marketing and capacity building through various campaigns and workshops. USAID through Abt Associates Inc., Danish International Development Agency

(DANIDA) and British Department for International Development (DFID) in particular provided financial and technical assistance to strengthen the implementation of the NHIS. The scheme also provides safety nets (premium payment exemptions for pregnant women, children under 18 years, indigents and the aged 70 years and above) which increased enrollment for the poor and vulnerable. Other distinguishing features of the NHIS that contribute to its success are: the comprehensive benefit package (95% of all diseases and health conditions in Ghana are covered) (NHIA, 2009), user portability, multiple providers and flexible choice of providers.

Competition among Districts

Finally, there was competition among district schemes to show success at annual review meetings which engendered them to embark on mass registrations on particular days of the month and the use of commission-based community registration agents to register people from house to house.

CHALLENGES TO WATCH

The gate-keeper arrangement in the Ghana health delivery system requires patients to first visit the lowest unit of health care (the CHPS compound) for basic out-patient services before they could be referred to the next level of health care- the health center, in that order up to the teaching hospital as the last stage, usually for complicated or specialized health cases. The ineffectiveness and the non-compliance to the gate-keeper system has unintended cost implications for the NHIS. This was a result of the insured shopping from provider to provider in search of better quality health care; all these billed the NHIS for reimbursement of claims, thus, increasing the claims bills. Effective gate-keeper policy and implementation systems are needed in the Ugandan health financing system to forestall any anticipated provider-shopping for health care.

Cost-Drivers of the NHIS

The main challenges that Ghana's NHIS is facing in terms of costs and leakages to the scheme as discussed in the previous sections could serve as red flags for any country, including Uganda which needs to adapt a similar NHIS model and its implementation strategies. Interviews with the NHIS management and stakeholders of the NHIS revealed these key cost drivers of the schemes which threaten its financial sustainability: fraud, adverse selection, providers and insured moral hazards, collusion between NHIS staff and providers to cheat the system. Other additional ones increase enrollment and increased health care claims, huge premium-exempt categories, huge administrative cost and leakages (corruption) and fee-for-service provider payment method.

CONCLUSION

This chapter has outlined the health care financing reforms in Ghana on the pathway towards universal health coverage. Among its peer countries in the Sub-Saharan Africa, Ghana's NHIS is a beacon for health care financing. However, there is still room for improvement of the scheme despites its phenomenal achievements.

The NHIS presents useful lessons for peer-countries in their quest for the establishment of a single-payer national health insurance scheme. Ghana's NHIS is a classic case of an experiment for Africa. Key factors that promoted the growth of Ghana's NHIS were: strong political will, existing community solidarity, prevailing poor conditions of health care and high out-of-pocket payment of health care, the learning by doing approach, the legal framework, predominant tax funding and generous health care benefits package. Other success factors include existing decentralized local government system, political stability, and development partnership in the implementation of the NHIS.

Challenges of the NHIS are predominantly health care provider fraud, inefficiencies in fund management, adverse selection of members due to huge premium exempt categories, increased utilization and financial sustainability challenges. The scheme has adopted innovative ways of addressing some of the challenges notably, the introduction of instant biometric registration identification card, and verification devices, electronic claims submission, safety nets for the poor and vulnerable, value added tax national health insurance levy, G-DRG and capitation payment methods and portability of health care with active insurance membership. Also, the NHIS has a mix of both private and public health care providers who provide health care services for members of the NHIS. We learned from Ghana's NHIS model that, countries do not need huge resources or gold standard plan before establishing a universal health insurance. A combination of appropriate legislation, a tax funding mechanisms and strong political will means countries could establish their universal health insurance schemes using the learning by doing approach while adopting corrective measures on its path to success since there is no perfect health insurance scheme. These useful lessons from Ghana's NHIS model could possibly be adapted for low-and middle-income countries, in a country and cultural specific context, on their paths towards universal health coverage.

REFERENCES

African Union. (2009). *Health Financing in Africa: Challenges and Opportunities for Expanding Access to Quality Health Care, Fourth Session of the African Union Conference of Ministers of Health.* Addis Ababa, Ethiopia 4th-8th May.

Agyepong, I. A., & Adjei, S. (2008). Public Social Polic Develo pment and Implementation: A case Study of the Ghana National Health Insurance Scheme. *Health Policy and Planning*, 150-160.

Anarwat, S. G. (2012). *Health Promotion in Northern Ghana: The Contribution of NGOs.* LAP Lambert Academic Publishing.

Anarwat, S. G. (2018). *Ghana's National Health Insurance Model: Advancing Financial Protection Equity of Health Care Access and Financial Sustainability (Ph.D. Dissertation).* Waltham, Massachusetts: ProQuest -Brandeis University.

Annie, S., Kumi-Kyereme, G., & Anarwat, S. G. (2001). *Quality Assessment of Mutual Health Organizations in Ghana.* Bethesda MD: Partners for Health ReformPlus, Abt Associates.

Asenso-Okyere, W. K., Osei Akoto, I., Anum, A., & Appiah, E. N. (1997). Willingness to Pay for Health Insurance in a Developing Economy: A Case Study of Households in Ghana Using Contingent Valuation Study. *BMC Health Services Research*, 7:114.

Atim, C., Grey, S., Apoya, P., Anie, S. J., & Aikins, M. (2001). *A survey of health financing schemes in Ghana.* Bethesda MD: Partners for Health Reformplus, Abt Associates.

Atim, C. (1998). *The Contribution of Mutual Health Organizations to Financing, Delivery, and Access to Health Care: Synthesis of Research in Nine West and Central African Countries.* Bethesda, MD: Partnerships for Health Reform Project, Abt Associates Inc.

Atim, C. B., & Sock, M. (2000). *An external evaluation of the Nkoranza community financing health insurance scheme, Ghana. Technical Report No. 50.* Bethesda, MD: Partnerships for Health Reform Project, Abt Associates Inc.

Basaza, R. (2015, October 21). *The NHIS in Uganda.*

Basaza, R., O'Connell, S. T., & Chapcakova, I. (2013). Players and processes behind the national health insurance: a case study of Uganda. *BMC Health Services Research*, 13-357.

Blanchet, N., & Acheampong, O. B. (2013). *Building on Community- based Health Insurance Schemes to Expand National Coverage: The Case of Ghana.* Bethesda MD: Health Finance and Governance Project (HFG) Abt Associates,

East African Community. (2014). *Situational analysis and Feasibility Study of Options for harmonisation of Social Health Protection systems towards Universal Health Coverage in the East African Community Partner States.* Arusha: East African Community.

Ghana Statistical Service - GSS, Ghana Health Service - GHS, and ICF International. (2014). *Ghana Demographic and Health Survey 2014, Final Report.* Rockville, Maryland, USA: GSS, GHS, and ICF International.

Government of Ghana Minstry of Health. (2014). *Annual Report.* Accra.

Government of Ghana, Ministry of Health. (2007). *Annual program of work (POW) 2007.* Accra: Ministry of Health.

Government of Ghana, Minsitry of Health. (2016). *National Health Insurance Scheme Technical Review Committee Reoport.* Accra: MOH.

Government of Ghana, Ministry of Health. (2004, August). *National Health Insurance Policy Framework -Revised Edition.* Accra: Ministry of Helath.

International Labour Organization (ILO). (2005). *Improving Social Protection for the Poor: Health Insurance in Ghana. The Ghana Social Trust Pre- Pilot -Project Final Report.* ILO.

Jehu-Appiah, C., Aryeetey, G., Spaan, E., & Agyepong, I. (2010). Equity and Efficiency feasibility of strategies to identify the poor: An application to premium exemptions under National Health Insurance in Ghana. *Health Policy*, 166-173.

Ministry of Health. (2010a). *Health Sector Strategic and Investment Plan 2010/11-2014/15.* Kampala: Ministry of Health: Government of Uganda.

Ministry of Health. (2015a). *Annual Health Sector Performance Report 2014/15.* Kampala: Ministry of Health: Government of Uganda.

Ministry of Health, Ghana. (2004, August). *National Health Insurance Policy Framework -Revised Edition.*

Nyman, J. (1999). The Value of Health Insurance The Access Motive. *Journal of Health Economics 18(2) 141-52, 18*(2), 141-152.

Nyonator, F., & Kutzin, J. (1999). Health for some? The effects of user fees in the Volta region of Ghana. *Health Policy Plan, 14*(4), 329.

Owusu-Sekyere, E., & Bagah, D. A. (2014). Towards a Sustainable Health Care Financing in Ghana: Is the National Health Insurance the Solution? *Public Health Research, 4*(5), 185-194.

Republic of Ghana. (2010). *National Health Insurance Scheme Annual Report (2010).*

Republic of Ghana, Ministry of Health. (2015). *Holistic Assessment of the Health Sector Programme of Work 2014.* Accra.

Saleh, K. (2013). *The Health Sector in Ghana: A comprehensive Assessment.* Washington DC: The World Bank.

Shieber, G., Cashin, C., Saleh, K., & Lavado, R. (2012). *Schieber, G., CashiHealth Financing in Ghana Direction in Human Development, The World Bank.* Washington DC: Direction in Human Development, The World Bank.

United Nations General Assembly. (2015). *Transforming our world: the 2030 Agenda for Sustainable Development,* New York: Resolution adopted by the General Assembly on 25 September 2015.

Waddington, C. J., & Enyimayew, K. (1989). A price to pay: The impact of user charges in Ashanti-Akim district, Ghana. *Int J Health Plann Manage*, 17-47.

World Bank. (2016, June 25). *Open data.* Retrieved from http://data.worldbank.org/: http://data.worldbank.org/country.

World Health Organization. (2011). *The Abuja Declaration, Ten years On.* Geneva: WHO. Retrieved from http://www.who.int/healthsystems/publications/abuja_report_aug_2011.pdf?ua=1.

World Health Organization. (2016). *Ghana Fact Sheets of Health Statisitics 2016, Africa Health Observatory.* WHO Regional Office for Africa.

Yeboah, Y. (2003). *Partnerships in Health Service. Prospects and Challenges in Ghana.* Dortmund: SPRING Research Series.

In: The Journey …
Editors: Robert Basaza et al.
ISBN: 978-1-53618-323-8

Chapter 8

WHAT ARE THE KEY LESSONS OF THE JOURNEY TO UNIVERSAL HEALTH INSURANCE COVERAGE? A MEASURED QUANTITY, QUALITY AND TYPES OF REFORMS MAY BE NECESSARY

***Robert Basaza*[1,2,*] *and Prossy K. Namyalo*[3]**
[1]Gudie Incubation Centre, Kira Municipality, Uganda
[2]Uganda Christian University Mukono MPHL Program,
[3]Ndejje University, Faculty of Social Sciences, Uganda

INTRODUCTION

This chapter focuses on the possible ways forward with health financing and establishment of universal health insurance coverage in Uganda. It also provides what LMICs with similar level of development like Uganda could

* Corresponding Author's E-mail: rbasaza@gmail.com.

consider for adoption. A measured quantity, quality and types of reforms may be necessary.

HEALTH FINANCING

At the current level of public health financing of US$ 10 per capita against the WHO recommended level of US$ 84 and funding level of 7% of the government budget [1], Uganda has to search out-side the box for better ways of improving the status quo. In line with Kutzin health financing reforms and universal health coverage models, no single health financing mechanism or health financing reform can suffice [2]. Uganda like other countries facing similar challenges will need to employ a mix of health financing mechanisms and sector reforms. The country will have to step up the speed of introducing contributory health insurance mechanisms, introduce user-fees for a section of people and modify the current state of abolition of user-fees. Decentralization of health facilities or district services to the extent that accountability remains at the point of usage or health facility will have to be strengthened. Private public health partnership has to be fully explored. The health workforce will need motivation as the single most central driving intervention based on a realistic dialogue. Incentives for health workers have to be built and regularly reviewed. Managed healthcare competition has to be put in place as applicable. Uganda and other LMICs have to make a deliberate effort to raise their budget provisions, in particular African countries could make appropriate steps to commit 15% of their budgets to healthcare in line with the Abuja declaration. Health economic efficiency measures need to be applied. These could include the principle of "gate keeping" where facilities at the lowest level are used first before attending higher level facilities. It has to be established and enforced through statutory instruments. Separation of demand and supply sides of healthcare will have to be established. Shepherd et al., points out that cost analysis of services has to be regularly carried out so as to inform policy and practice [3]. Investments' on determinants of health which include domestic and personal hygiene, housing, clean water, nutrition, food and moreso "continuity of care" will have to be fully explored and established.

National Health Insurance Scheme

The state and related actors have to place the establishment of the National Health Insurance (NHIS) on must to do list. Building a critical mass of knowledgeable actors and social marketing will need to be at the heart of implementation. The use of policy stream phenomenon where actors have to focus on tabling the problem, the proposal and politics at play may accelerate the realization of the scheme [4]. The world success stories on establishment of social health insurance schemes in Ghana and Rwanda emanate from key commitment and the centre stage at highest level of government in realization of their political agenda. The role of a champion in policy realization process is always pivotal [5].

Keys Lessons for Uganda and Other LMIC

What are the key lessons for Uganda and other LMIC countries to adopt in realization of universal health insurance coverage?

Political Will

A key factor in the success of a universal health insurance coverage is a strong political will behind the implementation of the NHIS. In Ghana for example, the government then in power, was determined to have the NHIS succeed in order to retain power in the subsequent elections (NHIS was a campaign promise of a major political party). Also, the government adopted a multifaceted and all-involving marketing approach that included social mobilization and marketing; community mobilization; local and national media campaigns; civil society, workers' unions, NGOs, and Ministry of Health involvement at the national and grassroots levels. Moreso, there was use of renowned religious and traditional leaders to voice the NHIS message in their jurisdictions.

Uganda and other LMICs, in quest for developing their national health insurance, can draw on both the positive experiences and challenges of Ghana NHIS to ignite the implementation process in their country-specific contexts. The experience in Ghana showed that high-level political commitment, popularity of the proposed reform, and sound technical analysis may be insufficient to avoid implementation difficulties. The political party and the then president's support was a key success factor in Ghana. The then ruling party and president also wanted to show the electorate that their party had fulfilled an election pledge before the next elections. Rwanda's success has been a function of the president's direction to increase access to health care for every citizen as a way of the regimes legitimacy based on rapid socio-economic development [6]. Greater attention and focus needs to be placed on recognizing, analyzing, and managing the political interests of key stakeholders during the policy process.

Mix of Financing Sources

Uganda and other LMICs will have to explore use of multiple sources of meeting premiums in realization of universal health insurance. Key among them is employer-based contributions directly or through NSSF (2.5% payment from the social security fund in Ghana), taxation (2.5% VAT from Ghana) [7] and donor contributions (Global Fund in Rwanda). A framework has to be put in place so that all the residents can enroll into the scheme despite the financial ability.

Decentralization of the Schemes

The district focus in the path to universal health insurance in Ghana and Rwanda has been key in increasing coverage and local ownership by the contributors. There has been central support in training the scheme operators to ensure correct interventions and operations.

Learn by Doing

The National Health Insurance Scheme – Rashtriya Swasthya Bima Yojana (RSBY) in India was introduced in several states by the Prime Minister with the aim of improving poor people's access to quality healthcare. As often happens with complex schemes, delays and challenges may arise. Not everything was perfect: at the beginning, the scheme was hardly operational and many hospitals complained of lack of training and delays in the reimbursement of their expenses. Some evaluators suggested a road map should have been prepared in advance: The first problem was coordination between the various departments entrusted with the implementation of the scheme; the second was the need for improvement in RSBY. The third issue was the capacity of staff to use appropriate technology, and fourth; the issue of misaligned incentives [8]. There is no perfect design before the launching of any scheme. Learn by doing also comes out clearly in the case of Ghana and Rwanda as well. Kutzin further adds that no single instrument or scheme can be "the answer." Most important is what are key questions and issues to help countries move towards dynamic, learning, adaptive systems. No reform instrument is inherently good or bad. It depends on context and the nature of the problem that a country is trying to solve. Most importantly, reforms should be oriented to objectives: what problems are we trying to solve? An informed public debate about particular reform options needs to be preceded by a process to gain consensus on the nature of the problems that need to be solved and thus the objectives of reforms [2].

Launch a National Health Insurance Scheme from Existing Schemes

Low and Middle-income Countries would benefit from experiences and practices of existing micro-health insurance schemes as they grapple with national coverage. This was the experience in Rwanda, Ghana and Thailand among others.

REFERENCES

[1] Ministry of Health. 2017. *National Health Accounts Report.* Ministry of Health Kampala, Uganda.

[2] Kutzin, J. 2012. Health Financing Policy Division, WHO. *Presentation at Satellite Session, 2nd Global Symposium on Health Systems Research*. Beijing, China.

[3] Shepard, D. S., Hodgkin, D. and Anthony, Y., 1998. *An Analysis of Hospital Costs: A Manual for Managers*. Geneva: World Health Organization.

[4] Béland, D. and M. Howlett. 2016. The Role and Impact of the Multiple-Streams Approach in Comparative Policy Analysis. *Journal of Comparative Policy Analysis: Research and Practice*, 18:3, 221-227, doi: https://10.1080/13876988.2016.1174410.

[5] Basaza, R., A. Kinegyere, A., Sewankambo, N. 2018. A national framework for sustainability of health knowledge translation initiatives in Uganda. *International Journal of Technology Assessment in Health Care. Cambridge University;* 34(1) 1-9. Accessible from: http://dx.doi.org/10.1017/S0266462317004482.

[6] Chemouni, B. 2018. The political path to universal health coverage: Power, ideas and community-based health insurance in Rwanda. *World Development*; 106:87-98.

[7] Jehu-Appiah, C. 2011. Equity aspects of the National Health Insurance Scheme in Ghana: Who is enrolling, who is not and why? *Soc Sci Med*; 72(2):157-65.

[8] Thakur, H. 2015. Study of Awareness, Enrollment, and Utilization of Rashtriya Swasthya Bima Yojana (National Health Insurance Scheme) in Maharashtra, India. *Front Public Health*; 3: 282. Accessible on 28 February 2018 from: https://www.ncbi.nlm.nih.gov/pmc/articles/PMC4703752/citedby/.

About the Editors

Robert Basaza [MBchB (MAK), MSc-HE (York, UK), PhD (Ghent)] is a Professor of Public Health and Health Economics. He has taught at various Universities: Uganda Christian University, St. Augustine International University, Clarke International University, Makerere and Kyambogo Universities. He has research, consultancy and publication experience in Africa and Europe in health insurance. His research interests are health economics and financing and, other health systems.

Prossy Kiddu Namyalo [PGD M&E (UMI), MA HMPP (Leeds, UK)] is a Public Health Expert and Lecturer at Ndejje University. She prior worked with Health Insurance Programs for several years. She has been involved in designing, promoting, implementing, managing and research of health insurance.

Chrispus Mayora [MA Econ (MAK), MHEC (Queensland), PhD Fellow (Wits)]. Lecturer and Health Economist at Makerere University School of Public Health, Uganda. Has vast teaching, research and consultancy experience in the fields of Health Economics, Health Financing, Costing, Economic Evaluations in Health, Health Systems Performance Assessment and Private sector in Health.

Donald S. Shepard [B.A., M.P.P and Ph. D Harvard University] is a Professor at the Schneider Institutes for Health Policy, Heller School for Social Policy and Management, Brandeis University, MA, USA. His work focuses on health insurance, cost-effectiveness analysis, incentives, and health financing, with studies in Uganda, other LMIC and USA.

Proofread by: Eric Nelson Haumba [BIS (UCU), CPD (Pretoria), MScIS (MAK)] is Chief Librarian and Lecturer at YMCA Comprehensive Institute Kampala. He has interest in interdisciplinary research: ICT4D, Knowledge Management, Information Ethics, Library Automation and Digitization, Health Informatics, Open Access, Intellectual Property, Agro-Ecology and Community Advocacy.

INDEX

A

B

C

D

E

F

G

H

I

P

Q

R

S

T

W